Clinical Techniques in Ophthalmology

Commissioning Editor: Michael Parkinson
Project Development Manager: Lulu Stader
Project Manager: Frances Affleck
Designer: Stewart Larking

Published with the support of AMO (Advanced Medical Optics)

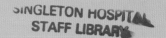

Clinical Techniques
in Ophthalmology

Edited by

Simon N Madge MA MRCP MRCOphth
Specialist Registrar
West of England Eye Unit
Royal Devon & Exeter Hospital
Exeter
UK

James P Kersey MA MRCOphth
Specialist Registrar
Department of Ophthalmology
Norfolk & Norwich University Hospital
Norfolk
UK

Matthew J Hawker BMedSci (Hons) MRCOphth
Specialist Registrar
Department of Ophthalmology
Norfolk & Norwich University Hospital
Norfolk
UK

Meon Lamont MB ChB MRCOphth
Senior House Officer
Department of Ophthalmology
Southampton General Hospital
Southampton
UK

Illustrations by Meon Lamont

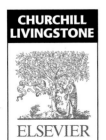

CHURCHILL
LIVINGSTONE

ELSEVIER

Edinburgh   London   New York   Oxford   Philadelphia   St Louis   Sydney   Toronto 2006

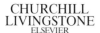

CHURCHILL
LIVINGSTONE
ELSEVIER

An Imprint of Elsevier Limited

© 2006, Elsevier Limited. All rights reserved.

The rights of Simon Madge, James P Kersey, Matthew J Hawker and Meon Lamont to
be identified as editors of this work have been asserted by them in accordance with the
Copyright, Designs and Patents Act 1988

First published 2006

ISBN 10: 0443 103046
ISBN 13: 978-0-443-10304-9

British Library Cataloguing in Publication Data
A catalogue record for this book is available from the British Library

Library of Congress Cataloging in Publication Data
A catalog record for this book is available from the Library of Congress

ELSEVIER your source for books,
journals and multimedia
in the health sciences

www.elsevierhealth.com

The
Publisher's
policy is to use
**paper manufactured
from sustainable forests**

Working together to grow
libraries in developing countries

www.elsevier.com | www.bookaid.org | www.sabre.org

ELSEVIER   BOOK AID
             International   Sabre Foundation

Printed in China

Foreword

It gives me great pleasure to write the foreword for this book which addresses the need to explain to neophyte ophthalmologists the basic principles in a way that clarifies rather than confuses.

As a very junior ophthalmologist I was made aware of the sheer volume of knowledge about the subject when I asked my consultant how I should prepare for the DO exam. He replied that I should read Duke–Elder's twelve volumes … twice!

Since those days, the cumulative knowledge base has increased exponentially but trainees *still* fail exams because they cannot do a cover test, have trouble explaining the concept of astigmatism to a patient and cannot calibrate a tonometer. This highlights the need for a book that starts at the beginning and explains the principles first, which, when understood, provide a firm foundation for all that additional knowledge to come. In these pages you will find almost every aspect of ophthalmology covered, from writing up notes to understanding refractive surgery techniques, and from mastering biometry to the basics of ocular therapeutics; subjects that will also be relevant for other healthcare professionals.

Ophthalmology is extraordinarily complex, both technically and clinically, and induces bewilderment in the uninitiated when presented with a slitlamp or a page of orthoptic notes. This book seeks to unravel those mysteries and cover the whole range of ophthalmic examination skills, procedures, investigations and instruments that will be faced by the trainee in those first years of mastering the subject. Happily, at that stage in their careers, the process is made easier by an insatiable desire for knowledge that is fuelled by enthusiasm for one of the most satisfying branches of medicine!

This is a book written by trainees for trainees. The style is refreshing, the explanations clear and the advice practical. Tips and pitfalls reflect those gems that have been passed down from generation to generation of ophthalmologists. The authors have accumulated and condensed a wealth of information together with beautiful diagrams and illustrations … and if you are no longer a trainee, it will do no harm to go back to the beginning again and read this book!

Nick Astbury
President, The Royal College of Ophthalmologists
June 2005

Acknowledgements

We are extremely grateful to the following:

Karen Mills, Martyn Buxton-Hoare, Paula Hughes and the staff of Advanced Medical Optics for their support from the book's beginnings.

Michael Parkinson, Lulu Stader and Geraldine Craig for their publishing and editorial input.

Fran Hazelwood, Maggie Vaughan and Joy Smith for being willing model patients.

Norfolk & Norwich Hospital Neurophysiology Department for their help in procuring some of the images in the electrodiagnostics chapter.

Duckworth & Kent Ophthalmic Equipment Company.

Roger Baer for his encouragement at the time of the book's beginnings and Peter Simcock for his encouragement and advice near its completion.

Ali, Caroline, Selina and Sarah for their understanding, patience and unending support over the last two years.

SNM
JPK
MJH
ML

Preface

The purpose of this book is to provide a general introduction to some of the concepts and skills that are a prerequisite to being a competent and useful junior ophthalmologist. It has been assembled from the knowledge of fellow ophthalmologists, who are still close enough to the beginning of their careers to remember the need for both clarity and simplicity of explanation. The various chapters include concise but clear introductions to clinical optics, basic ophthalmic surgical procedures including phacoemulsification, investigations that are routinely requested by juniors and an introduction to ophthalmic drugs. In addition, this book also contains several suggested schema for examining patients, which should suffice for most postgraduate Examinations as well as the ophthalmic clinic.

Most, if not all, available textbooks in ophthalmology assume a level of understanding of ophthalmological examination techniques, equipment, investigations and procedures, which is never formally taught. Unlike in medical school, where hours are devoted to mastering different examination routines and learning the ins and outs of the stethoscope, the new junior ophthalmologist often has to pick up skills essentially by osmosis. Where clinical texts abound, there are few easily accessible and practical handbooks for basic clinical skills in ophthalmology. This is where we hope you will find this book essential reading.

The various chapters are carefully designed to be read individually (cross-references will direct the reader elsewhere if necessary), in sections (e.g. optics, surgical procedures, examination routines, etc.) or, if desired, from front to back. Included in the text are numerous boxes providing extra information for the interested reader and data such as suggested settings for laser procedures, which the reader may need to refer to throughout his or her career. Throughout the book, numerous clear and colourful illustrations will help you understand the principles involved.

Although written primarily with trainee ophthalmologists in mind, this book has been designed to be as accessible as possible to other healthcare professionals. It is hoped that all those working in the field of ocular health will find this book helpful in explaining the many concepts and techniques that abound in this fascinating speciality.

May 2006

SNM
JPK
MJH
ML

Contributors

Morag Adams BSc (Hons) MB ChB
Senior House Officer
Department of Ophthalmology
Musgrove Park Hospital
Taunton, UK

Paul Baddeley MA MRCOphth
Specialist Registrar
Department of Ophthalmology
University Hospital of Wales
Heath Park
Cardiff, UK

Matthew J Hawker BMedSci (Hons)
MRCOphth
Specialist Registrar
Department of Ophthalmology
Norfolk & Norwich University Hospital
Norfolk, UK

James P Kersey MA MRCOphth
Specialist Registrar
Department of Ophthalmology
Norfolk & Norwich University Hospital
Norfolk, UK

Thomas LNH Kersey MRCOphth
Senior House Officer
Princes Charles Eye Unit
Windsor, UK

Meon Lamont MB ChB MRCOphth
Senior House Officer
Department of Ophthalmology
Southampton General Hospital
Southampton, UK

Simon N Madge MA MRCP MRCOphth
Specialist Registrar
West of England Eye Unit
Royal Devon & Exeter Hospital
Exeter, UK

Bill McDermott BSc (Hons) RN
Ophthalmic Nurse Specialist
Department of Ophthalmology
Musgrove Park Hospital
Taunton, UK

S Vasant Raman MS FRCS
Specialist Registrar
Royal Eye Infirmary
Plymouth, UK

Richard Sidebottom BM BCh
Senior House Officer
Department of Ophthalmology
Musgrove Park Hospital
Taunton, UK

Contents

Section 1
Basic clinical optics

1

Emmetropia, ametropia and presbyopia

SN Madge

Introduction

Spectacles, lenses and optics have successfully baffled junior ophthalmologists for many years. In the UK at least, optics is usually picked up by osmosis over a couple of years before being met as a formal requirement in the optics and refraction section of the MRCOphth Examinations. Optometrists, in contrast, have the benefit of a full degree course in the subject and are taught the subject properly. This section of the book is not designed as an alternative to the popular optics and refraction textbooks that are available; it is, however, hopefully more accessible and is designed to introduce the relatively difficult concepts in a friendly and simple manner.

An understanding of the concepts introduced in the following chapters will be more than sufficient to allow you to deal with the refractive issues that routinely confront junior ophthalmologists. Furthermore, you are very likely to impress your seniors if you have a good grasp of this complex subject early in your career.

Emmetropia and accommodation

The eye acts as a set of lenses, focusing light onto the retina. If a patient's relaxed eye is of the correct shape, the light coming from a distant source is focused clearly onto the retina and the eye is said to be *emmetropic* (essentially 'normal-sighted', with clear distance vision). A distant source is technically defined as at infinity, but 6 or more metres is usually a good approximation, and from such a distance emerging light rays are assumed to be parallel with one another (Fig. 1.1A). In order to see clearly objects that are closer than infinity, whose light rays are actually slightly divergent, the focusing power of such an eye must increase—this is called accommodation.

The majority of the focusing of the eye (*refraction*) occurs in the cornea, while the remainder is in the lens. The cornea is not thought to be capable of changing shape significantly and so any dynamic changes in the power of the eye's focusing abilities are due to alterations in the lens. Although the exact mechanism remains unclear, when the ciliary muscle contracts, the lens moves forward to a degree and also becomes slightly thicker, increasing its refractive power and so allowing closer objects to be seen. The reason that closer objects need more refractive power to be seen is that their emerging light rays are diverging and not parallel as from a distant object (Fig. 1.1B). Obviously, there must be a limit as to how much the lens can accommodate in this fashion, which defines the *near point* of the eye: the shortest distance that the object can be from the eye while remaining in focus.

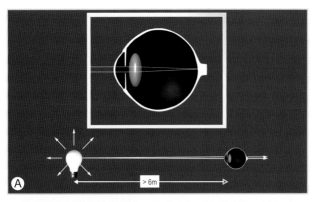

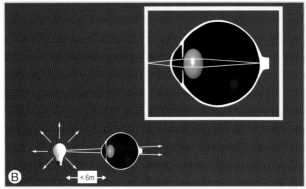

Fig. 1.1 Emmetropia and accommodation. A. Light rays from a source further than 6 m away are deemed parallel and are focused by the relaxed emmetropic eye on the retina. **B.** Light rays from an object nearer than 6 m are divergent and need a stronger (thicker) lens to focus the image on the retina.

Presbyopia in emmetropia

The amount that an eye can accommodate reduces with age, a phenomenon known as presbyopia, which is related to changes in lens proteins and the supporting zonules. With other factors being equal, this means that the relaxed emmetropic eye will see distant objects just as clearly aged 10 as when aged 70, but will have a markedly reduced near point in older age.

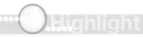

Highlight

Correction of presbyopia

To compensate for the loss of lens power for viewing near objects, older emmetropes wear 'reading glasses' to help them see such objects more clearly. These are simply additional positive ('*plus*') lenses to replace the refractive power lost from the poorly accommodating, ageing human lens. As patients age, progressively higher power lenses are required for near vision, as less and less accommodation is available. In the case of a patient who has undergone conventional cataract surgery, no accommodation remains and such patients are totally dependent on relatively high-powered spectacles for near activities.

The basic pathophysiology in presbyopia starts as soon as the first year of life, but is not clinically significant in emmetropes until around the beginning of the fifth decade. *Cycloplegic eyedrops*, such as tropicamide, simulate presbyopia in younger patients, affecting visual acuity for near vision far more than for distant vision; the accommodating mechanism of the eye is paralysed with such medication.

Ametropia—myopia and hypermetropia

The relaxed emmetropic eye is able to focus distant light rays clearly on the retina; for an emmetrope, the *far point* is therefore said to be at infinity. If a differently shaped, relaxed eye has more or less refractive power than an emmetropic eye, parallel light rays from distant objects will not be focused on the retina and the image seen will be blurred, a condition known as ametropia (either long- or short-sighted).

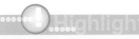

Myopia

If a relaxed eye has more refractive power than the emmetropic eye (Fig. 1.2), it is known as *myopic*, otherwise referred to as 'being short-sighted', which ranges from mild (practically emmetropic) to severe (see below). In myopes, even when the ciliary muscles are relaxed, the eye is too powerful to see distant objects clearly as the eye is effectively focused for a closer distance. So-called 'low' myopes might well be able to see clearly objects up to 2 m away with no accommodation, but struggle to see more distant objects well (e.g. road signs), which are beyond their far-points. 'High' myopes, however, might struggle to see anything clearly beyond 10 cm (far point), and with active accommodation might be able to see clearly as close as 5 cm (near point).

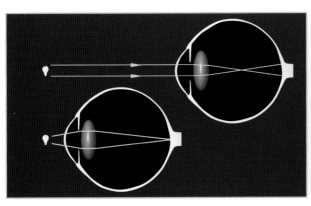

Fig. 1.2 Myopia. Light rays are brought to a focal point in front of the retina in a myopic eye (top). Nearer objects are focused on the retina (bottom). Note the lens is not accommodating in either image. Spectacles are therefore needed to see distant objects.

Basic clinical optics

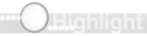

Hypermetropia

Hypermetropia is the opposite of myopia and is slightly more difficult to understand. In this condition, the relaxed eye is so shaped that parallel light rays from distant objects are not focused enough by the refractive structures of the eye. In other words, the eye's power is too weak and the rays would come to a focus behind the eye (Fig. 1.3). The relaxed, young *hypermetropic* eye is, therefore, unable to see distant objects clearly but is fortunately able to accommodate, which increases the effective power of the eye, allowing parallel rays of light to be focused on the retina. Hypermetropic eyes, therefore, usually have good distance vision (albeit while accommodating) and are hence known as 'long-sighted'.

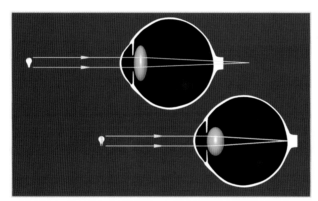

Fig. 1.3 Hypermetropia. The weak focusing power of a hypermetropic eye causes light from distant objects to focus behind the retina (top). However, accommodation will increase the refractive power of the eye (bottom), and the image will be brought to focus on the retina.

Unlike myopes, who have blurred distance vision, many young hypermetropes may not be aware of their condition because in most cases the requisite accommodation occurs subconsciously. It is only when eyestrain from excessive accommodation develops (due to prolonged near work) that the condition manifests itself. However, as presbyopia becomes more advanced with age, there comes a point when the accommodation required to see distant objects clearly is insufficient for the hypermetrope's requirements. At this stage, spectacles will need to be worn to see anything clearly, either in the distance or close-up.

Presbyopia in ametropia

The basic pathophysiological process in presbyopia occurs at the same stage in emmetropes, myopes and hypermetropes. However, it becomes manifest at different stages in each condition. For example, by the time an emmetrope is 40 years old, his accommodation will have reduced to the point where he might feel more comfortable with spectacles for reading, but his distance vision will of course be unaffected. A 40-year-old low myope, in comparison, might have functional (but, by definition, not perfect) distance vision. However, because his eyes' far-points are closer than infinity (as per the emmetrope), his accommodation, although reduced, is sufficient to provide him with clear reading vision; it might be another 10 years or so before such a patient requires reading glasses. Depending on the severity (degree) of hypermetropia, a 30-year-old hypermetrope may require reading glasses to see close objects clearly, although he will probably have sufficient accommodation in reserve to see distant objects clearly at that stage in his life. While wearing no spectacle correction, *presbyopia therefore tends to affect hypermetropes before emmetropes, who are affected before myopes*.

Clinical ametropia

SN Madge

Further concepts in ametropia

After the last chapter, it should now seem obvious that it is vital to consider every patient's refractive state in effectively two dimensions:

1. What is the degree and type of ametropia (i.e. is the patient myopic or hypermetropic and by what degree)?
2. How much accommodation does the patient have available (i.e. what is the functional focusing range, bearing in mind the ametropia and degree of presbyopia)?

The *dioptre* (D) is the international optometric unit that is used to classify patients' ametropia and range of accommodation. A +1 D *spherical* lens is the power of lens required to focus parallel light to a point, at a distance of 1 m from the lens (in such a case, the *focal length* of the +1 D lens would be 1 m). The power of the lens is the reciprocal of the focal length in metres; thus, for example, a +8 D lens has a focal length of 12.5 cm.

In clinical optics, we often talk about the patient's 'refraction'; in fact, this is an abbreviation for 'refractive correction', because an eye is always described in terms of the correction required for that eye to become emmetropic, not the power of the eye itself.

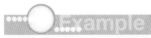 Example

Refractive correction

A myopic (or short-sighted) eye is more powerful than an emmetropic eye, meaning that parallel light is focused to a point in front of the retina. In order to make the myopic eye emmetropic (and have clear distance vision), *minus* lenses (that diverge the light rays) must be used, and the patient's refractive correction will therefore be something like '−1 D' (low myopia) or '−8 D' (relatively high myopia). In hypermetropia, the power of the eye is too low and additional *plus* lenses are required. These positive lenses effectively help the uncorrected hypermetrope's ciliary muscles, allowing clear, relaxed distance vision, on top of which the patient's normal accommodation can then be exerted to see nearer objects if required (Fig. 2.1).

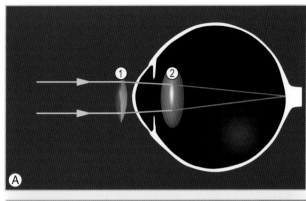

Fig. 2.1 Refractive correction. A. If the appropriate convex (*plus*) lens (1) is placed in front of a hypermetropic eye, the distant light rays are converged sufficiently for the weak crystalline lens (2) to bring the image into focus on the retina. **B.** If the eye now accommodates, the increased refractive power of the crystalline lens (2) will bring diverging light rays from near objects into focus on the retina.

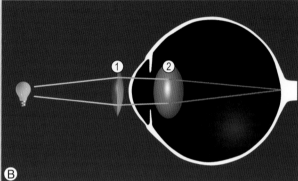

Knowing a myope's refractive correction allows you to work out the far point; in metres, this is simply the reciprocal of the dioptric correction. In the case of a −3 D myope, the far point will be $\frac{1}{3}$ m, or 33.3 cm, meaning that such a patient can avoid the effects of presbyopia simply by removing spectacles to read. Any degree of hypermetropia produces a far point that is beyond infinity (usually referred to as behind the eye, as this is where the light rays would focus); the '+' correction represents the amount of positive dioptres of lens needed to give a new far point of infinity. In a young patient, this '+' correction is equivalent to the amount of accommodation needed to give clear distance vision, e.g. +5 D.

In the absence of accommodation (e.g. advanced presbyopia, cycloplegia or after cataract extraction), myopes will have clear vision at their far point, as will emmetropes (distant objects), but hypermetropes will have no clear vision without spectacles. This is of great relevance during cataract extraction, when the power of the intraocular lens (IOL) implant can be varied. In this common scenario, where patients have no effective accommodation, there is no refractive advantage to creating a low hypermetrope (too weak an IOL implant), whereas creating a low myope will usually be very satisfactory if emmetropia cannot be guaranteed.

Other aspects of ametropia

Hypermetropic eyes

- Generally short (axial hypermetropia) in terms of their axial length.
- Shallow anterior chamber, which predisposes to a narrow drainage angle and an enhanced risk of angle closure glaucoma.
- Shallow anterior chamber also makes cataract surgery more challenging.
- Crowded optic discs may enhance risk of ischaemic optic neuropathy.

Myopic eyes

- Generally long (axial myopia) in terms of axial length: may predispose to needle stick injuries during anaesthesia.
- High myopes are more likely to suffer retinal detachments and macular degeneration.
- A very deep anterior chamber (high myopes) can make cataract surgery challenging.

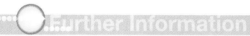 Further Information

Aphakia

Aphakia (absent lens) is an extreme form of hypermetropia. With the eye's native lens removed, previously emmetropic eyes are often about +12 D hypermetropic, which clearly requires powerful spectacles to be corrected. Sadly, such spectacles have many optical problems associated with them, especially in unilateral aphakia (an example of anisometropia), and such patients often rely on contact lenses to provide reasonable sight. Of course, a high myope who becomes aphakic might actually lose the perfect amount of refractive power (through losing the lens) to become emmetropic. All aphakic patients, of course, have no accommodation and therefore rely on different spectacle lenses for near vision.

3

Astigmatism

SN Madge

Introduction

The eye is not a perfect sphere. In many cases, the cornea is more steeply curved in the vertical meridian than the horizontal, meaning that the eye is effectively slightly 'squashed' from above. An increased curvature of the cornea in the vertical meridian means that the eye is optically more powerful in this meridian than the horizontal. Consequently, as light rays enter the eye, light in the vertical meridian is focused anteriorly to light in the horizontal, creating a 'blur circle' near the retina. This inequality in focusing between meridians represents astigmatism (Fig. 3.1).

Astigmatism usually arises from disparities in the different meridia of the cornea, but may in fact also be due to differing refractive powers (again in different meridia) within the lens of the eye (*lenticular astigmatism*). In addition, a subluxed intraocular lens implant may also produce refractive powers that are unequal in different meridia, so too producing astigmatism.

Regular or irregular astigmatism?

Where the angle between the maximum and minimum meridia of curvature is 90 degrees, the astigmatism is termed *regular*; in the vast majority of patients, this is the case. After corneal grafts, trauma and in conditions such as keratoconus, the meridia of curvature are far from perpendicular and the term *irregular astigmatism* is applied.

Where the refractive power is greater in the vertical meridian than the horizontal, the astigmatism is termed *with-the-rule*, and in the converse situation *against-the-rule*. Interestingly, the eye changes shape during life, often first exhibiting with-the-rule astigmatism before sometimes developing against-the-rule astigmatism in later years. Some eyes exhibit astigmatism that does not conform to these simple horizontal/vertical rules but which is still regular; such eyes exhibit *oblique astigmatism*, which is amenable to correction in the same way as other types of regular astigmatism, but with lens powers (at 90° to each other) away from the horizontal and vertical meridia.

Correction of astigmatism

As for myopia and hypermetropia, lenses can be produced that correct this 'over-focusing' in one meridian only. Such lenses are termed *cylindrical* if only one meridian needs correction to produce emmetropia for the eye. If neither

Basic clinical optics

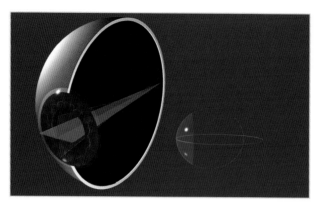

Fig. 3.1 Astigmatism.
If the corneal curvature is steeper (smaller radius of curvature, as illustrated in red) in one meridian than another (greater radius, as illustrated in blue) then the eye is said to have (corneal) astigmatism.

meridian is capable of focusing light rays on to the retina, then a *toric* lens will be required; such a lens has a different power in each meridian, with the final result being that all light rays from a distant object entering the eye are focused on the retina.

Corrective lenses for astigmatism are described in terms of their power (as per spherical lenses; p. 8) and their axis (a way of defining the meridian in which the lens power is exerted, see below). In the case of regular, with-the-rule corneal astigmatism, as the cornea is more powerful in the vertical meridian, lenses can be introduced to either reduce the power in this meridian or alternatively increase the power in the horizontal meridian. In either case, the power in both meridia would then be equal; the choice regarding which would be the best option depends on the underlying ametropia of the eye and also the personal preference of the practitioner.

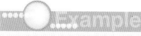 **Example**

Cylindrical lenses

If a patient was −1 D myopic in the vertical meridian (i.e. with-the-rule astigmatism: vertical corneal meridian steeper than horizontal) and emmetropic in the horizontal meridian, then a −1 D cylindrical lens with power acting in the vertical meridian would result in emmetropia (remember the −1 refers to refractive correction and not the eye itself). Similarly, a +1 D lens with power acting horizontally would neutralise the astigmatism but would result in the eye being −1 D myopic in all meridia.

Power and axis of a cylindrical lens

Cylindrical and toric lenses cause confusion because their notation is notoriously difficult to understand. Although their power is described using the dioptre as

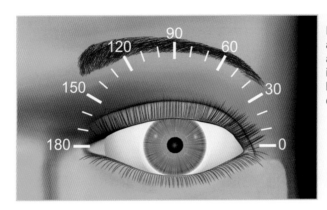

Fig. 3.2 The axis of astigmatism. Described as shown in the figure, irrespective of whether the left or right eye is being considered.

above, *their angle of action is represented by the axis of the lens, which is always at 90 degrees to the actual power exerted by the lens.* Thus, in order to correct the astigmatism in the example above, a –1 D lens with axis horizontal (and therefore power vertically) will be required; alternatively, a +1 D lens with axis vertical (and therefore power horizontal) would result in the eye being –1 D myopic in all meridia as above, but having no astigmatism (no difference in power between meridia). Remember, cylindrical lenses have no power in the meridian of their axis.

Angles (in degrees) are used to define the direction of the axis and run from 0° to 180°, with 0° and 180° both being horizontal, 90° vertical, and running from right to left anticlockwise as the practitioner looks at the patient in either eye (Fig. 3.2). In regular astigmatism, as there are only two astigmatic axes, an axis of, for example, 210° is equivalent to 30° (210° –180°) and is always referred to as such.

Plus or *minus* cylinder?

Returning to the above example of with-the-rule astigmatism, it will now become clear that the eye can be represented by two different, but equivalent prescriptions:

1. A cylindrical lens of –1 D with axis horizontal is written as: 0.00/–1.00 × 180. In other words, for such an eye, 0 D power is required to produce emmetropia after the –1 D cylindrical lens with axis 180° has been added.

2. A cylindrical lens of +1 D with axis vertical will produce an eye that is –1 D myopic in all meridia. To neutralise this, a further lens of –1 D will be required in addition to the cylinder to produce emmetropia. Such a combination of lenses is written: –1.00/+1.00 × 090. In other words, –1 D power is required to produce emmetropia after the +1 D cylindrical lens with axis 90° has been added.

The lenses 0.00/–1.00 × 180 and –1.00/+1.00 × 090 are equivalent as they both lead to emmetropia. The first prescription is an example of using *minus cylinder*, whereas the second is using *positive cylinder*. Both represent with-the-rule astigmatism.

Basic clinical optics

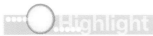

With- or against-the-rule?

- With-the-rule astigmatism: *minus* cylinder axis at 180°, or positive cylinder axis at 90°.

- Against-the-rule astigmatism: positive cylinder at 180°, or *minus* cylinder axis at 90°.

Only remembering one of these four possibilities will allow you to simply classify astigmatism, as you can transpose the prescription given to you into your favoured form (see below).

Most practitioners develop a preference for using either positive or *minus* cylinders early in their careers, but it is possible to convert one prescription to the other fairly easily. This is called transposition.

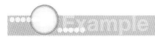

Transposition

- To convert 0.00/−1.00 × 180 to positive cylinder form, add the spherical lens (0) to the cylindrical (−1) to produce the new sphere (−1). Change the sign of the original cylinder (−1 becomes +1) and subtract or add 90° to the axis (180° becomes 90°).

- To convert −8.00/+3.00 × 165 to *minus* cylinder form, −8 added to +3 equals −5 (new sphere); the +3 cylinder becomes −3 (new cylinder power) and the axis changes from 165° to 75° (165 − 90 = 75). The new prescription is therefore −5.00/−3.00 × 075.

Further concepts in astigmatism

SN Madge

Astigmatism and the cornea: *k* readings

An additional source of confusion in this topic arises from *k* readings (keratometer, p. 66) and their relationship to optical prescriptions. In order to successfully prescribe contact lenses or calculate the requisite power of IOL after cataract surgery, it is necessary to measure the amount of corneal curvature in different meridia and derive an estimation of the corneal astigmatism (bearing in mind that the lens may also be responsible for some astigmatism). The keratometer gives a *k* reading (in dioptres) of the power of each corneal meridian measured. To understand the relationship between such measurements and optical prescriptions, it is vital to remember that such prescriptions are the refractive corrections required to produce clear distant vision for the eye as a whole, and are not necessarily an accurate reflection of corneal curvature per se.

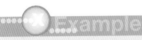

Corneal *k* readings

Taking our original example of with-the-rule astigmatism (0.00/–1.00 × 180): if this is entirely corneal in origin, then the vertical corneal meridian will be steeper than the horizontal and the *k* reading will be 1 D greater in the vertical meridian than the horizontal, e.g. 43 D vertically and 42 D horizontally.

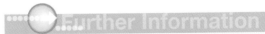

Advanced example of *k* readings

Taking the prescription –5.00/+3.00 × 180 (against-the-rule), one would expect that the *k* readings would be greater for the horizontal meridian than the vertical. If the *k* readings were in fact 43 D horizontally and 44 D vertically (with-the-rule *corneal* astigmatism), then it implies that the astigmatism is actually due to a structure other than the cornea—usually the lens—and in this case is contributing 4 D of astigmatism (3 D from the prescription plus 1 D of with-the-rule corneal astigmatism neutralised).

Basic clinical optics

Astigmatism and corneal instrumentation

Any surgical procedure performed on the eye has the potential to alter the eye's refractive correction. For example, in astigmatic keratotomy, incisions are deliberately made in the cornea to alter the degree of astigmatism of the eye. Non-corneal surgery also has its effects; retinal encirclement by a buckle (as in retinal detachment surgery) usually leads to slight elongation of the axial length and hence induces an increase in myopia.

Corneal incisions and sutures

- Incisions in the cornea (usually ≈90% of corneal thickness in astigmatic keratotomy) tend to flatten the cornea in that meridian, especially if combined with another incision diametrically opposite, so reducing the refractive power in that meridian. The site of the incision in routine phacoemulsification is also often placed to reduce astigmatism in this way.

- A suture placed in the peripheral cornea, if tight, will tend to increase the refractive power in that meridian, especially if combined with a further suture diametrically opposite.

- After a corneal graft, sutures are often left in situ for long periods of time. If there is found to be a great deal of astigmatism, then removal of diametrically opposite sutures (only) tends to flatten the cornea in that meridian, so reducing the refractive power in that meridian.

Where to make the incision or remove the suture?

In the absence of lenticular astigmatism, the following examples are true:

- In with-the-rule astigmatism, such as +3.00/+2.00 × 090 (equivalent to +5.00/−2.00 × 180), the steeper corneal meridian is the vertical. A superior incision, so flattening the cornea, is therefore the approach of choice in order to reduce the corneal astigmatism in this case.

- In against-the-rule astigmatism, such as +3.00/+2.00 × 180 (equivalent to +5.00/−2.00 × 090), the steeper corneal meridian is the horizontal. The incision of choice is therefore a temporal one in this case. It should be noted, however, that temporal incisions affect the corneal astigmatism less than superior incisions because the corneal limbus (and hence site of incision) is further from the optical axis temporally than superiorly.

However, it is impossible to accurately predict the varying contributions of lenticular and corneal astigmatism, and the site of incision should be chosen on the basis of keratometry readings and not the spectacle prescription.

- In a post-corneal-graft eye, the refractive correction may be −4.00/−4.00 × 060. In such a case, the steepest corneal meridian is at 150° (90° to the minus cylinder prescription, or in the line of the positive cylinder correction) and the sutures to be removed are in this meridian, i.e. 4 o'clock and 10 o'clock as one looks at the eye. It would, however, be preferable to obtain either keratometry or corneal topography to confirm the refractive state before intervening.

The common theme in all these examples is to flatten the cornea (incision or suture removal) on the axis of the positive cylinder. Conversely, a compression suture should be placed in the line of the axis of the negative cylinder.

Further classification of astigmatism

The following terms are often found in Examinations:

- *Simple myopic astigmatism:* one meridian is emmetropic and the other myopic.
- *Simple hypermetropic astigmatism:* one meridian is emmetropic and the other hypermetropic.
- *Compound hypermetropic astigmatism:* both meridia are hypermetropic but by differing amounts.
- *Compound myopic astigmatism:* both meridia are myopic but by differing amounts.
- *Mixed astigmatism:* one meridian is myopic and the other is hypermetropic.

Spherical equivalent

This is an important concept, widely used in optics, to determine the predominant refractive correction of an eye in the face of astigmatism. It also represents the spherical prescription most likely to give the clearest vision (if astigmatism must be neglected—often for audit (!) purposes). To calculate the spherical equivalent, simply halve the cylindrical part of the prescription and add it to the spherical part.

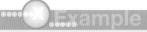 Example

Spherical equivalents

Take a prescription +1.00/–5.00 × 130. The spherical equivalent is therefore $(+1) + (-5/2) = -1.5$ D. Therefore, a lens of strength –1.5 D would give the clearest vision if cylindrical lenses are not to be considered. The spherical equivalent is the same regardless of the form of the prescription: +1.00/–5.00 × 130 in positive cylinder notation is –4.00/+5.00 × 040. The spherical equivalent of this is also –1.5 D $(= (+5/2) + (-4))$.

Lenses and their identification

SN Madge

Although a focimeter (p. 62) offers relatively quick, accurate spectacle identification, it is not always available, and there are some other very simple techniques that can be used to gain much information about a patient's spectacles.

Myopic or hypermetropic?

Gross ametropia can be easily spotted, regardless of the material of the lens. Look at the patient with the spectacles on (Fig. 5.1). Compare the line of the lateral margin of the face above and below the lens with that within the lens.

- Hypermetropia requires convex lenses for correction, which also produce magnification; the line seen within the lens is therefore lateral to the line outside.
- Myopia requires concave lenses for correction, which produce minimisation; the line seen within the lens is therefore medial to the line above and below the lenses.
- If the line within the lens is practically continuous with that outside, then low myopia or low hypermetropia is expected.

The only exception to these rules is in mixed astigmatism, when rotation of the lens through 90° will produce the opposite result.

Is an astigmatic correction present?

Look at a cross through the lens. Rotate the lens. If there is any distortion ('scissoring') of the target while rotation occurs, then astigmatism is present; otherwise the lens in question is spherical.

With and *against* movements

In the case of spherical lenses, movement of a spectacle lens while looking through it at a target will identify the type (Figs 5.2 and 5.3).

- Apparent movement of the target *with* the direction of lens movement is due to a concave (*minus*) lens, whereas apparent movement of the target *against* the direction of lens movement is due to a convex (*plus*) lens.

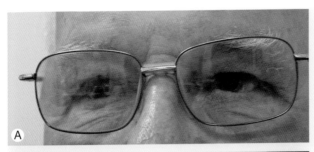

Fig. 5.1 Myopic or hypermetropic.
A. Hypermetropic corrections (magnifying) exaggerate the line of the temple laterally through the spectacle lens. **B.** Myopic corrections (minimising) move the line of the temple medially through the spectacle lens.
C. Virtually emmetropic corrections produce no significant effect on the line of the temple through the lens.

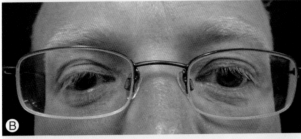

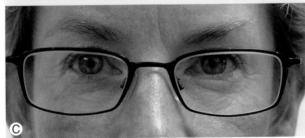

In simple cylindrical lenses, there will be no apparent movement of the target if the direction of lens movement is along the axis of the lens.

- If the direction of movement is perpendicular to the axis, then apparent movement of the target will occur *with* in a negative cylinder and *against* in a positive cylinder.

In toric lenses, the direction of apparent movement depends on the power of the lens in the meridia considered.

Example

Toric lens identification

In the case of the toric lens −3.00/+4.00 × 180, because the cylindrical component (4 D) has its axis at 180°, there will be no cylindrical power in this meridian. Any apparent movement of the target while moving the lens along this axis will be entirely dependent on the spherical (−3 D) component, and thus the movement seen will be *with*. For movement along the 90° meridian, we must consider both the spherical (−3) and the cylindrical (+4) components, which total +1 D; the apparent movement seen will therefore be *against*.

Basic clinical optics

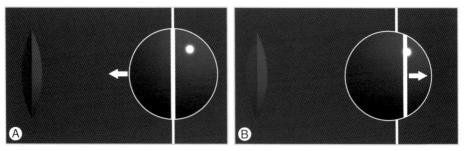

Fig. 5.2 Convex lens identification. A. A convex (*plus*) lens produces a magnified image (white line). If the lens is now moved in the direction of the arrow, the image will move in the opposite direction (image B). **B.** The convex lens has been moved to the left and the image of the white line moves in the opposite direction.

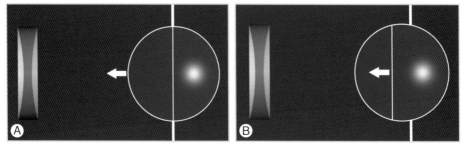

Fig. 5.3 Concave lens identification. A. A concave (*minus*) lens produces a diminished image (white line). Moving the lens in the direction of the arrow will result in the image moving in the same direction (image B). **B.** The concave lens is moved to the left and the image of the white line moves even further in the same direction.

Non-refractive considerations

- *Lens form.* Is the lens single vision, bifocal or progressive (varifocal) in nature? Bifocals are easy to spot; some difficulty exists in separating single vision lenses from progressive lenses. To spot a progressive lens, view a target through the upper portion of the lens; while maintaining fixation on the target, rotate the lens upwards to look through the lower portion. If the lens is progressive, magnification of your fixation target will be observed.

- *Lens markings.* Progressive lenses will often carry a marking (e.g. '+2.00') on the lens itself, visible by holding the lens up to the light. This represents the add correction incorporated into the lens from distance portion to near.

- *Glass or plastic?* Should be obvious from weight and sound when tapped.

- *Colour?* Should be obvious, but photochromic lenses may of course appear clear in dark environments; however, they darken with age. An anti-reflective coating may often be seen by oscillating the spectacles under a light—purple reflections are seen.

- *Is there a prism in the lens?* See below.

Prisms

Prisms deviate light but have no refractive power themselves. They are used to control diplopia but must be used with caution, as injudicious use can lead to asthenopic symptoms (eye strain). A focimeter can help you to identify prisms, but in its absence it is important to be able to detect a prism and identify its direction of action.

Stare at a target and then move the lens into and out of your line of sight. Is the target displaced when the lens is in your line of sight, regardless of the position? If so, then it is likely that there is a prism in the lens. A prism deviates light towards its base, which actually means that an image (through the prism) is deviated towards its apex. The direction of target displacement seen is therefore in the direction of the prism apex and may be horizontal, vertical or both. *Bear in mind that when it comes to notation, prisms are always defined in terms of their base and not their apex.*

The power of a prism is usually expressed in either prism dioptres (Δ) or degrees (°), where 1 Δ is the strength of a prism that produces an apparent deviation of light by 1 cm at a distance of 1 m from the prism (with incident light parallel to the base of the prism). For ophthalmic use, one prism dioptre is approximately equivalent to $\frac{1}{2}$°.

Prisms can be incorporated into spectacles or can be added on externally for short-term treatment, as in *Fresnel prisms*. Fresnel prisms are thin plastic sheets containing tiny individual prisms that function as one large prism; they are often to be found stuck onto the glasses of patients exiting orthoptic departments. Interestingly, Fresnel prisms were originally used in old-fashioned lighthouses.

Spectacles and some uses of lenses

SN Madge

Wearing others' spectacles

In the absence of significant astigmatism, clear vision is possible through another person's spectacles in certain circumstances.

In the case of myopic corrections, the *minus* concave lenses diverge light rays, which stimulates accommodation (effectively simulating the process that occurs in uncorrected hypermetropia). Although prolonged use, especially for near objects, may lead to eyestrain, an emmetrope or low myope may use a slightly higher myope's spectacles with little difficulty, although minimisation of objects may be noticed.

Hypermetropic corrections are positive lenses, which converge light. As previously mentioned, such lenses effectively do the job of the ciliary muscles, allowing accommodation to relax. Thus, emmetropes are able to see near objects clearly through such lenses (as they will have to in later life when presbyopia develops). Myopes wearing *plus* lenses will find themselves more myopic, as their near point will be further reduced—although their accommodation will allow them to see clearly even closer than before.

Spectacles and strabismus

Childhood concomitant strabismus (or squint) is intimately related to refractive correction. Accommodation occurs simultaneously with convergence of the eyes and pupillary constriction. For each individual, there is a relationship between accommodation and convergence, the so-called accommodation:convergence (AC:A) ratio; with a high ratio, excessive convergence occurs for each dioptre of accommodation exerted.

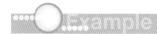

Strabismus

- A +5 D hypermetropic child needs to exert 5 D of accommodation to see distant objects clearly. In so doing, even with a normal AC:A ratio, convergence is stimulated and may lead to a convergent squint for distant objects, worse still with further accommodation for nearer objects.

- With a high AC:A ratio, even a mildly hypermetropic child may develop a convergent squint for near objects because too much convergence is stimulated.

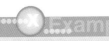 **Example**

Strabismus, cont'd

In both these examples, the use of *plus* lenses will relax accommodation and the drive for convergence will be reduced. In the first example (fully accommodative esotropia), a +5 D correction should correct the squint in the absence of amblyopia. In the second (convergence excess esotropia), bifocal spectacles (with more *plus* in the near segment) will relax accommodation and relieve excessive convergence for near.

Spectacle prescription notation

Errors in spectacle dispensing occur for many reasons; correct prescription notation is paramount to avoid such problems.

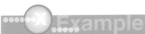 **Example**

Example: +4.50/−2.25 × 012 and *not* 4.5D/−2¼ × 12°

- Always ensure that the sphere is preceded by a plus or a minus sign; absence of the correct symbol is ambiguous.
- Ensure that the prescription for both eyes is in the same form, positive or negative cylinder.
- Omit the degree symbol (°); its inclusion has been mistaken for a zero. The same is true for the dioptre symbol (D).
- Write the axis of the cylinder in three figures, not two. This is standard practice.
- Use decimal points and ideally two decimal places, not fractions.
- Use clear handwriting!
- In the case of a near prescription as well as a distance prescription (usually presbyopia), write the additional plus required as e.g. 'add: + 2.50' for each distance prescription; this is invariably the same for both eyes.
- In the presence of a prism, ensure that the prism is prescribed for the correct eye and that the base (as well as the power in prism dioptres Δ) is specified: BO = base out, BU = base up, BI = base in, and BD = base down.

Biometry, emmetropisation and 'A' constants

SN Madge

Introduction

Ocular biometry for intraocular lens implantation during cataract surgery is still evolving. There has been a trend in recent years away from traditional ultrasound biometry towards partial coherence laser interferometry (e.g. the Zeiss IOLMaster) due to the ability to measure true foveal axial length, greater accuracy and reproducibility, albeit at currently greater expense. Greater accuracy is certainly desirable, as it gives patients a higher likelihood of visual success while minimising refractive surprises, a common cause of litigation in ophthalmology.

Overview

Regardless of the method employed, the goal of preoperative ocular biometry is to provide a set of data from which the postoperative spherical equivalent refractive correction can be estimated for a particular choice of intraocular lens (IOL) implant. Central to this calculation are two measurements: (i) the axial length and (ii) the average keratometry reading, as well as the 'A' constant specific to the intended IOL implant.

These data are then used in an empirically derived mathematical formula (e.g. SRK/T, Haigis, Hoffer Q, etc.) to provide an estimate of postoperative refraction for a given IOL power. Virtually all biometry machines will carry out this function automatically, providing a list of estimated postoperative refractive corrections for different IOL powers.

The differences between the different formulae are beyond the scope of this book, however, suffice it to say that it is common practice for different formulae to be used in different eye units and also for different formulae to be used for differing axial lengths (e.g. the Hoffer Q formula is often used for eyes of very short axial length). It is important to be aware of your local policy.

The measurements

There are a multitude of different machines available for both measuring the axial length and the corneal curvature (p. 66), all of which cannot be covered by this book. Please refer to individual manuals for instructions for use of such equipment.

Keratometry readings can be provided either in dioptres or millimetres (radius of corneal curvature). Two readings (highest and lowest curvatures) are usually supplied with axes, with the two readings being taken perpendicular to one another (in the case of regular astigmatism). (If only one reading is given by an automated keratometer, this can mean that the corneal surface being measured is a perfect sphere.) The mean of the two dioptric readings is then used in the chosen biometric formula. In the face of high or irregular astigmatism, it is very useful to study corneal topography prior to surgery.

Compare the keratometry readings with the refractive data available. Are the refractive data explained by the keratometry readings or is there a significant degree of lenticular astigmatism present (p. 15)? There may be important implications for the site of the incision.

With respect to the axial length, there are a number of important considerations prior to accepting the biometry as correct:

- Are the readings for the two eyes similar (e.g. within 0.2 mm of each other)? If not, do the available refractive data mirror the difference seen between the two eyes? If considering such data, it is important to use data obtained prior to the onset of significant nuclear sclerosis, as this may have induced a myopic shift.

- Ensure that the appropriate setting has been used for the eye in question; e.g. if the eye is aphakic, pseudophakic or filled with silicone oil, ensure that the relevant option has been selected on the machine.

- Ensure that the relevant biometric formula is being used for the axial length of the eye. Refer to local unit policy.

Target sphere (spherical equivalent) and consent

The biometry formulae only provide a solution for the postoperative spherical equivalent refractive correction. Astigmatism (and where to make the incision etc.) is dealt with elsewhere in this book (Ch. 4).

In most cases, aiming for a postoperative refraction of 0 D (emmetropia) will produce a satisfactory result. However, exactly 0 D is very rarely an option and usually one has to choose a target refraction in the region of +/− 0.25 D. For example, although a +0.2 D result is closer to 0 D than −0.25 D and might seem more desirable, in the absence of accommodation there is no refractive advantage in being rendered hypermetropic. Thus, in the absence of other considerations, the mildly myopic result is favoured (as at least perfect focused vision will be attained for one focal length without spectacles, as opposed to none at all if hypermetropic, as the far point is beyond infinity).

It is also vital to consider the other eye. If making one eye emmetropic will result in a difference of greater than ≈2 D between the two eyes, then symptomatic aniseikonia (differing image sizes in the two eyes) may result. Patients must be advised that second eye surgery may well be necessary in such a situation, even if there is no current second eye lens opacity. Alternative options in such a situation include:

- Aiming for a postoperative result similar (within ≈1.5 D) to the other eye, but this clearly precludes emmetropia in the future (common solution).

- Contact lens use in the other eye until second eye surgery becomes necessary.

Basic clinical optics

If aiming for emmetropia, particularly in a young patient, ensure that they are aware of the absence of accommodation. In other words, they will need spectacles for reading and all tasks requiring close vision.

Warn patients that although you are aiming for emmetropia, only a percentage of patients will achieve such a result (number dependent on local biometry service and audit). Due to astigmatism and minor errors in biometry, it is likely that a low spectacle prescription may be necessary to 'fine tune' postoperative vision, although most patients are perfectly 'functional' (without spectacles) for distance vision.

Although obvious, it is also important to warn patients that their spectacle prescription will change postoperatively.

Also consider the background ametropia:

- For example, low myopes often enjoy being myopic! The ability to read without spectacles is not to be sniffed at and many myopes undergoing cataract surgery wish to retain this ability. It is important to discuss the implications of emmetropisation to all such patients; although their unaided distance vision would obviously improve, they would be unable to read without spectacles, thread needles etc. Aim for a spherical equivalent close to their current refraction ($\approx$ −2.5 D ideal) if they want to be left myopic.

- Higher myopes may be more grateful for emmetropisation as they will tend to read with spectacles on; however, it is important to give them the option of a low myopic result.

- Try to ensure that myopes do not end up hypermetropic postoperatively, as they will have lost any refractive advantage that they had.

- Hypermetropes are generally easily satisfied, because even a slightly myopic result means that they can focus clearly on something without spectacles (as opposed to nothing preoperatively). Emmetropia is the ideal.

Also consider the health of the eye. In advanced macular degeneration, it can be a significant advantage to a patient to be left hypermetropic, as the resulting hypermetropic corrective lenses required lead to added magnification, which may be very helpful.

Beware the first eye result. It is often the case that the actual results of first eye surgery are far from the predicted results. If there is no obvious reason why this should be the case, it is then wise to:

- Warn the patient that a degree of unpredictability exists with respect to the second eye surgery.

- Adjust the biometry accordingly. For example, if the first eye ended up +1 D hypermetropic, use a more powerful lens than suggested by the formula to try and increase the likelihood of emmetropisation.

Monovision

Some patients function very well with one eye emmetropic and one eye $\approx$ −2.5 D myopic, reaping the benefits of clear distance vision with one eye and reading vision with the other, while seemingly being able to ignore disabling aniseikonia. This can be the result of careful preoperative planning in cataract surgery (in order to negate presbyopia), but it may be difficult to predict which patients will do well. A preoperative contact lens trial is suggested.

'A' Constants

An 'A' constant represents a correction (or 'fudge') factor in biometry formulae specific to the lens type used to achieve an accurate result. Widely inaccurate results are obtained if attention is not paid to 'A' constants.

Each IOL used will have a different 'A' constant; the easiest way of visualising what they mean is to consider that they reflect the anterior–posterior position of the IOL within the eye (Fig. 7.1). For example, an anterior chamber IOL may have an 'A' constant of 115.0, whereas a similar posterior chamber IOL may have a value of 118.0. The lower 'A' constant simply means that the IOL is sitting more anteriorly and therefore a lower powered IOL is required. With increasing 'A' constants, and thus effectively a more posterior IOL position, a higher power is required to achieve the same desired postoperative refraction.

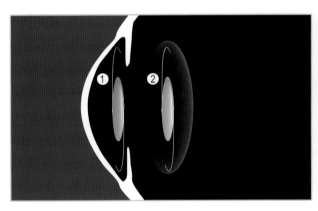

Fig. 7.1 IOLs and 'A' constants. A lens in the anterior chamber (1) has a lower 'A' constant than one that is placed in the capsular bag (2).

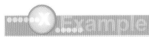

'A' constants

Example 1

An appropriate biometry formula suggests that an IOL (with 'A' constant 118.0) of +20.0 D is required to produce emmetropia. During the operation, you are informed that the only IOLs available are of 'A' constant 119.5. The IOL of choice to produce emmetropia in such a situation would be +21.5 D. (119.5 – 118 = 1.5, add this to +20.0 D to get +21.5 D).

Example 2

Your consultant ruptures the posterior capsule and wants to place an anterior chamber IOL ('A' constant 115.0). Preoperative biometry suggests that, for emmetropia, a +20.0 D IOL ('A' constant 118.0, posterior chamber IOL type) should be used. The appropriate anterior chamber IOL power is +17.0 D (118 – 115 = 3, subtract this from +20.0 D to get +17.0 D).

Basic clinical optics

The 'A' constants are initially set by the manufacturers for their specific IOLs. However, differing surgical techniques (between units and individual surgeons) may mean that IOLs may end up sitting in different positions, and it is recommended that continuous audit be undertaken to ensure that the manufacturers' 'A' constants are indeed correct for the local setting.

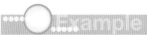

'A' constant audit examples

If postoperative audit reveals that spherical equivalent refractions are on average +0.8 D more hypermetropic than expected for a particular IOL, this can be interpreted as the IOL effectively sitting too posterior in the eye for its suggested 'A' constant. A locally implemented increase in the 'A' constant for that particular IOL should be applied, which will lead to more powerful IOLs being used and thus a move towards emmetropia (and myopia). This will explain in many units why the 'A' constants on the biometry printouts do not tally with the number on the IOL packaging.

Using the SRK/I formula

Suggested IOL Power = 'A' constant – 2.5 × (axial length mm) – 0.9
$$\times \text{(keratometry } k \text{ reading)}$$

Using an axial length of 20 mm and an average k reading of 47.78 D as examples (for such a short eye, the Hoffer Q equation would probably normally be used in clinical practice):

Suggested IOL 1 = 118.0 – (2.5 × 20) – (0.9 × 47.78)
$$= 118.0 - 50 - 43 = +25.0 \text{ D}$$

for emmetropia, but audit in the local eye unit reveals that this actually results in +0.8 D of hypermetropia! Therefore, increase 'A' constant by 0.8 to compensate. Thus:

Suggested IOL 2 = 118.8 – (2.5 × 20) – (0.9 × 47.78)
$$= 118.8 - 50 - 43 = +25.8 \text{ D}$$

for emmetropia. A repeat audit reveals that for these biometry figures, using a +26.0 D IOL (+25.8 not available) results in –0.2 D of myopia. Correction of the 'A' constant has been successfully applied.

Biometry in patients who have had refractive surgery

Detailed discussion of this topic is beyond the scope of this book. The problem in such patients is that standard keratometry makes assumptions that are not valid in an eye that has had a keratorefractive procedure. Data regarding the preoperative keratometry readings and pre- and postprocedural refraction are preferably all required, and also possibly corneal topography and a contact lens over-refraction.

8

Retinoscopy

SN Madge

Introduction

Retinoscopy provides objective measurements of the refractive state of the eye. In adults, these measurements are then often refined using subjective techniques to provide a final spectacle prescription (Ch. 11), but in children the retinoscopy data alone provide the basis for prescription. A solid understanding of basic clinical optics is a prerequisite for understanding the role and techniques of retinoscopy; it is suggested that this chapter be read in conjunction with the rest of the Basic Clinical Optics section.

This chapter will only deal with the *slit retinoscope* (as opposed to the slightly more unusual *spot retinoscope*, although the principles involved are similar).

Principles

The modern retinoscope consists of a light source, a mirror and a sight hole in the mirror, all arranged so that the observer, looking through the hole, can see whatever is illuminated.

The handle of the retinoscope has a cuff, which can be moved up and down. With the cuff down (preferred position), a condensing lens between the light source and the mirror allows diverging light rays to be emitted by the retinoscope. With the cuff up, the condensing lens is moved to such a position that converging light rays are emitted (Fig. 8.1).

Light entering the patient's eye is reflected by the retina and is then refracted according to the refractive state, before being viewed by the observer through the sight hole of the retinoscope.

Differing movements of the retinal light reflex are seen depending on the position of the cuff, the distance of the observer from the patient (*working distance*), the refractive state of the eye (i.e. emmetropic, myopic, etc.) and, of course, which way the retinoscope's light beam is moved.

By interspersing trial lenses between patient and examiner, *neutralisation* of the light reflex can be attained, which can then be easily converted into an objective measurement of refraction.

Although relatively simple, the actual optics of the retinoscope are beyond the scope of this book.

How to do it

- Turn the retinoscope on and place the cuff fully down. It will be noticed that the instrument emits a slit of light, which can be varied in its orientation by turning the dial of the retinoscope.

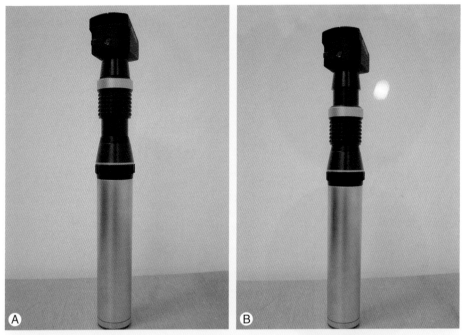

Fig. 8.1 Retinoscope. A. With the retinoscope cuff up, converging light rays are emitted. This position is not commonly used in retinoscopy. **B.** With the retinoscope cuff down (recommended position), diverging light rays are emitted.

- Place a trial frame on an adult patient. Dim the lights and ask the patient to observe the distant white spot of the light box. (The remainder of the chapter will concentrate on retinoscopy in ideal conditions, i.e. with no accommodation. For information on how to deal with accommodation and refracting real patients, see p. 42.)
- Position yourself carefully at the same level as the patient and at approximately arm's length (≈ 66 cm). Place your head so that it almost obscures the patent's view of the distant light source. Ask the patient to inform you if you do actually get in the way, as this will stimulate accommodation and cause spurious results.
- Look through the retinoscope while passing the slit across the patient's eye. After a bit of practice, you will begin to appreciate that as well as the slit being visible moving over the patient's eyelids and iris, there is also visible a further slit of light moving within the pupil.
- As for the direct ophthalmoscope, you will need to use your left eye to examine the patient's left eye, as well as your right for the patient's right eye.
- If this pupillary slit of light moves in the same direction as the slit of light seen on the external eye, the movement is described as *with* movement. If this pupillary slit of light moves in the opposite direction of the external slit of light, this is known as *against* movement (Fig. 8.2).
- When the cuff of the retinoscope is down, *with* movements necessitate the introduction of *plus* spherical lenses into the trial frame. *Against* movements require *minus* spherical lenses.

Basic clinical optics

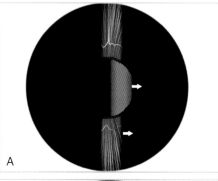

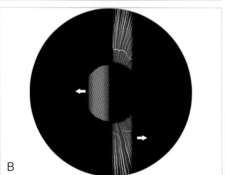

Fig. 8.2 Retinoscopy: *with* and *against* movements. A. A *with* movement is one where the retinal reflex moves in the *same* direction as the light beam of the retinoscope. **B.** An *against* movement is one where the retinal reflex moves in the *opposite* direction to the light beam of the retinoscope.

- As the progressive addition of lenses nears the correct prescription for the patient, the apparent speed of movement of the pupillary slit of light increases, as does the brightness of the reflex. (If the patient is highly ametropic, the speed of movement of the slit at the start of retinoscopy can be very slow indeed.)

- By titrating the movements of the slit with the trial lenses, there should come a point when neutralisation occurs. At this point, instead of seeing a pupillary slit, the entire pupil will fill with light and the reflex will appear very bright.

- At this point, note the lens in the trial frame and make a mental note of the distance you were from the patient when neutralisation occurred (working distance).

- Also note the direction (0–180°, see Fig. 3.2, p. 13) in which you were sweeping (moving) the retinoscope; this will be perpendicular to the light slit per se. For example, if neutralisation occurred when the light slit was vertical (90°, as in Fig. 8.2), the movement of the slit was in the horizontal direction (0° or 180°). In retinoscopy, it is the direction of retinoscopic slit sweep (and not the position of the light slit per se) that is recorded, along with the power of lens required for neutralisation (in a *power cross*, see below).

- Now try rotating the slit by 90° and trying again. If there is a difference in lenses required (for neutralisation) in these different axes, then it is possible that the patient has a degree of astigmatism.

- In the face of significant astigmatism, it may be noted that in most meridia of slit, the external light slit and pupillary slit are not orientated the same way.

  - Rotate the slit beam until the pupillary slit and external slit are perfectly orientated; this orientation represents one of the (two) axes of astigmatism and will be crucial for obtaining correct neutralisation, and also obtaining the correct prescription.

  - After finding the neutralisation point in this meridian, try rotating the slit through 90° and, after ensuring that the slit orientations match, find the new neutralisation point.

- To convert retinoscopy data into spectacle prescriptions, the working distance must also be taken into account (see below).

Working distance, power crosses and spectacle prescriptions

The notation of spectacle prescriptions and retinoscopy results (the power cross) is unfortunately inherently confusing. While spectacle prescriptions consist of the axes of lenses, it must be remembered that the power of a lens is actually at 90° to this axis (p. 13) and the power is what is measured by retinoscopy. Retinoscopy results are traditionally written in the form of a power cross, where a line is drawn for each of the two lens powers at the neutralisation point (lines therefore perpendicular to each other, forming a cross), with each line being orientated for the direction of retinoscopy *sweep* where neutralisation occurred. See below for an example.

The working distance correction (in dioptres) that must be applied to retinoscopy data is simply the reciprocal of the working distance in metres, which is then always *subtracted* from the data to provide the retinoscopy result.

For example, at a working distance of 66 cm, it was found that neutralisation occurred with −3 D in the trial frame while sweeping in the 180° meridian (light slit axis therefore at 90°), and with +1 D while sweeping in the 090° meridian (perpendicular to first reading). What is the retinoscopy result (power cross) and consequent spectacle prescription?

The reciprocal of the working distance (0.66 m) is 1.5. This is then subtracted from the retinoscopy result to give the answers:

- In 180° meridian, retinoscopy result = −3 − (1.5) = −4.5 D
- In 090° meridian, retinoscopy result = +1 − (1.5) = −0.5 D

The power cross is shown in Figure 8.3.

In terms of a spectacle prescription for this patient, there are two components requiring correction: first a cylindrical component of 4.0 D (the difference between the two lenses) and a residual spherical correction (either −0.5 D or −4.5 D, depending on whether *plus* or *minus* cylinder notation is used).

To convert these measurements into a spectacle prescription, remember that the power of cylindrical lenses acts at 90° to their axis. Thus, working in *minus* cylinder, the spectacle prescription needed is −0.50/− 4.00 × 090. To expand on this, the difference between the two lenses is 4.0 D (−0.5 − (−4.5)), whose power is exerted at 180° (and therefore of lens axis 090) and which is superimposed on the base sphere of −0.5 D. The same result transposed into *plus* cylinder form is −4.50/+4.00 × 180.

As an aside, if shorter arms necessitated a lower working distance of 50 cm, the reciprocal of 0.5 m is 2 and 2 D would be subtracted from each result rather than 1.5.

Basic clinical optics

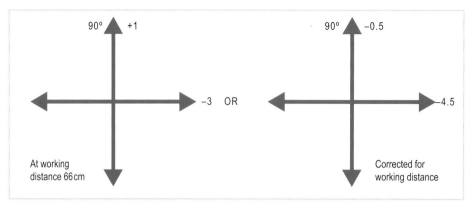

Fig. 8.3 Power cross diagrams. Summarising the findings of: retinoscopic neutralisation occurring with −3 D in the trial frame while sweeping in the 180° meridian (light slit axis therefore at 90°), and with +1 D while sweeping in the 090° meridian, at a working distance of 66 cm.

Can you go straight to the spectacle prescription without drawing a (confusing) power cross?

Yes—and outside of Examinations, this is pretty much standard practice when refracting adult patients.

It is possible to leave the first neutralised meridian's lens in place while retinoscoping the second meridian. In this case, you can use cylindrical lenses to measure the second meridian, which will save time in determining the spectacle prescription:

- With the first meridian (preferably the least *minus* or most *plus*) neutralised by spherical lenses, turn the slit through 90° and start placing cylindrical lenses in the trial frame so that their axis matches that of the slit. With the cylindrical lens in this position, its power (which is at 90° to the axis) will therefore be acting in the same direction as your new retinoscopic sweep direction.
- Add progressively stronger or weaker lenses according to the pupillary slit movement.
- At the second neutralisation point, the spectacle prescription will be the spherical lens (corrected for the working distance) *plus* or *minus* the cylindrical lens with the axis it is sitting in within the trial frame.

Troubleshooting

- *'The battery's fine, but the reflex is very dull.'* It is possible that you are retinoscoping a high myope or hypermetrope. Try interposing a −10 D or +10 D lens and having another go.
- *'I can't seem to get an end point (neutralisation point).'* Is the cuff down? Try asking a more senior ophthalmologist to demonstrate an end point to you.

- *'My results are far more "minus" than they should be.'* It is likely that your patient has been accommodating—you may have noticed swirling reflexes during retinoscopy. Ask the patient to keep staring at the light source, avoid putting your head in the way and ensure that the patient is adequately fogged from the outset (p. 42). Alternatively, consider a cycloplegic refraction (e.g. using cyclopentolate).

- *'My results are far more "plus" than they should be.'* Ensure that you have remembered to correct for your working distance and that you have *subtracted* it from the total and not added it.

9

Maddox rod

SN Madge

Introduction

This is a series of usually red, strong convex (*plus*) cylindrical lenses mounted together side-by-side as a trials lens. Its main use is in the measurement of extraocular muscle imbalance (described below), which is often a final step in refraction (p. 42).

Principles

Light from a distant point source (producing parallel rays of light) is viewed through the Maddox rod. Light passing through the cylindrical lenses in the same meridian as the axis of each cylinder passes through without refraction, thus remaining undeviated. The light in this meridian is focused by the eye itself, which produces a single line on the retina, perpendicular to the axis of the cylinders.

Light rays in meridia other than the cylinders' axis are converged by the powerful lenses to a point focus just in front of the eye, which is too close to be appreciated by the eye; thus, no image is seen.

In the testing of extraocular muscle balance, the Maddox rod is placed in front of one eye, while the other eye simply stares at the same distant light source. As the two eyes are actually seeing different images, a white spot and a red line (albeit both emanating from the same source), there is no stimulus to visual fusion and nothing to keep the two eyes from drifting apart except for the underlying tone of the extraocular muscles. The eyes are thus *dissociated*. Measuring the subjective distance between the two images with prisms thus allows a measure of extraocular muscle balance and an estimate of the degree of *phoria* of a patient (see 'Cover testing', p. 113).

How to do it

- Dim the lights.
- Give the patient his or her distance prescription to wear, mounted on a trial frame.
- Place the Maddox rod in the right (**r**od on **r**ight eye) front trial frame slot, with the cylinders running vertically to start with (axis vertical).
- Ask the patient to look at the white spot of the light box.

- The patient should start to appreciate a horizontal red line with the right eye. If not, momentarily occlude the left eye until the line is seen.

- Ask the patient whether the line that they see is level with, above or below the white spot of the light box. If level, this implies no vertical muscle imbalance (or *phoria*). If the line seen is above the spot, this implies a right *hypophoria*, and may be corrected by the introduction of prisms either base up on the right eye or base down on the left. If below the spot, this implies a right *hyperphoria*, correctable with prisms base down on the right or base up on the left. (Always put the base of the prism in the direction that you would want the eye to move to correct the situation.) Try introducing small prisms to align the red line and spot.

- Then, turn the Maddox rod through 90° so that the cylinders are now running horizontally. A vertical red line should now be appreciated.

- Ask the patient whether the red line is level with, or to the left or the right of the white spot. If level, there is no horizontal phoria. If the red line is to the left of the spot, an *exophoria* is implied, which can be corrected with base-in prisms in front of either eye. If the red line is seen to the right of the spot, an *esophoria* is implied, which can be corrected with base-out prisms in front of either eye. Try introducing small prisms to bring the red line and spot into alignment.

 Further Information

Further uses of Maddox rods

- Two Maddox rods can be used together (one in each eye) to provide an estimate of *torsional phoria*.

- Occasionally useful in hysterically blind patients.

Cross-cylinders

SN Madge

Introduction

Cross-cylinders ('cross-cyls') are often used in refraction. They are initially extremely confusing, but are exceptionally elegant methods of refining a cylindrical prescription. They are often referred to as Jackson's cross-cylinders, after the man that originally popularised their use (Edward Jackson, 1893–1929).

Design

Cross-cylinders are available in several different powers (commonly 0.5 D, 1.0 D and 2.0 D), but the basic principle is identical in each. Each cross-cylinder consists of a toric lens, where the power of the cylinder incorporated is twice that of the sphere, but of the opposite sign (Ch. 3). *Thus, the spherical equivalent of any cross-cylinder is always zero.* For example, a 0.5 D cross-cylinder would consist of a +0.25 D base sphere with a –0.5 D cylinder incorporated into it; this, of course, is identical to a –0.25 D base sphere with a +0.5 D cylinder incorporated into it (but just transposed). With this latter fact in mind, it should now become apparent that in any cross-cylinder, there is an axis of positive cylinder and an axis of negative cylinder orientated perpendicularly (Fig. 10.1).

The most elegant part of the cross-cylinder is the way that the handle of the instrument relates to the axes of the lens. The handle meets the lens midway between the two axes (i.e. 45° to both the positive and negative cylinders), which is very useful for refraction (see below).

Cross-cylinders in action

The use of cross-cylinders requires asking the patient to make forced choices between two options. If one option is preferred, the relevant changes are made and the patient is then given another forced choice to make. If both options are equally poor, then the end-point has been reached. This method is true for both axis and power verification—see below.

Minus or plus cylinder?

In refraction, first decide whether you are working in *plus* or *minus* cylinder. Most optometrists work in *minus* cylinder (e.g. prescriptions of the form +2.50/–3.50 × 175 or –0.50/–2.75 × 134 etc.), and therefore this is how examples will be presented below.

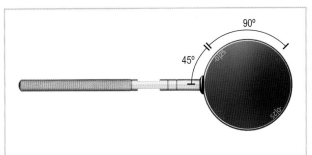

Fig. 10.1 Cross-cylinders. The axes of the positive and negative cylinders are at 90° to each other. They are both at 45° to the handle.

Checking the axis (Fig. 10.2)

In order to check a proposed axis of astigmatism in a patient (found by retinoscopy or from a previous spectacle prescription), simply hold the cross-cylinder so that its handle lies along the proposed axis (Ch. 11).

- Ask the patient whether they think the cross-cylinder makes the 'O' (see Ch. 11) look rounder (but not necessarily clearer) in this position ('position 1'), or whether it is rounder with the cross-cylinder flipped through 180° around the axis of its handle ('position 2', i.e. turned over, but keeping the handle in line with the axis).

- If the proposed axis of astigmatism is correct, then the patient will have no preference for more negative cylinder in either direction: both options will be undesirable.

- If the proposed axis is not coincident with the true astigmatic axis, then the patient should prefer the position of the cross-cylinder where the negative cylinder offered lies nearer the true negative axis. Thus, rotate the negative cylindrical lens (in the trial frame) towards the preferred negative axis of the cross-cylinder.

- Then repeat the process until no preference is expressed for the two positions of the cross-cylinder; this should be approximately the correct axis of negative cylinder.

Using cross-cylinders to establish the axis

In the absence of a retinoscope or previous prescription, the axis of astigmatism may also be established using a cross-cylinder.

- While asking a patient to fix on a round target, hold up the cross-cylinder and ask whether the patient finds the target rounder with the cross-cylinder in that position ('1') or whether they find the target rounder with the cross-cylinder rotated through 90° (position '2').

- Whichever position is preferred is a rough approximation to the location of the '−' cylinder and a '−' cylindrical trial lens (of similar power to the cross-cylinder) can be inserted in this direction, before proceeding with fine tuning of the axis as outlined above.

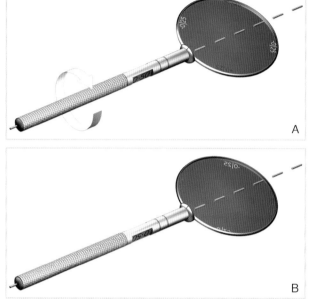

Fig. 10.2 Checking the axis. A. Position '1'. When checking the axis, the handle is held on the proposed axis (broken line) and the cross-cylinder then rotated through 180° (see diagram B). **B.** Position '2'. The handle is still positioned on the proposed axis, but the negative and positive cylinders have changed position.

A

B

Checking the power of the cylindrical correction (Fig. 10.3)

When the astigmatic axis has been established, the cross-cylinders can also be used to verify the requisite power of the cylinder.

- With the patient fixing on a large 'O', hold up the cross-cylinder with the '+' of the cross-cylinder in line with the proposed astigmatic axis (i.e. handle at 45° to the axis).

- Ask the patient if the 'O' looks clearer (not rounder) with the cross-cylinder in this position (e.g. '3') or when the cross-cylinder is flipped through 180° around the axis of its handle (e.g. 'position 4').

- If they prefer position '3', then reduce the '–' cylinder (equivalent to adding '+'); if they prefer '4', then increase the '–' cylinder.

- If the two positions are equally undesirable, then an end-point has been reached.

If refracting, adjust the sphere for the new cylinder

Remember to adjust the sphere in the trial frame if large changes to cylindrical power are made (Ch. 11). The reason for this is that, as mentioned above, cross-cylinders have a spherical equivalent of zero, whereas cylindrical lenses (in trial lens sets) do not; their spherical equivalent is half that of the cylinder. Adding a cylindrical lens will therefore change the overall spherical prescription in an undesirable manner, unless properly accounted for.

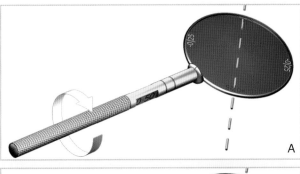

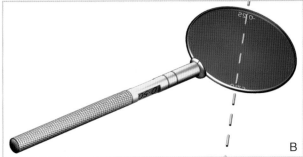

Fig. 10.3 Checking the power of the cylindrical correction. A. Position '3'. When checking the power of the cylinder, the proposed axis is held at 45° to the handle, and rotated through 180° (see diagram B). **B.** Position '4'. After rotating the cross-cylinder through 180°, the offered cylinder is changed from positive to negative.

Recheck the axis if you change the power of a cylinder

If a change of cylinder power is necessary, the new cylindrical lens can often be placed (accidentally) slightly off the recently established axis. Particularly with higher-powered cylindrical corrections (> 1 D), recheck the axis prior to fine tuning the power again. This may seem to add an unnecessary step to the routine, but it will probably pay dividends in the long term.

A suggested scheme for refraction

SN Madge

Introduction

The following scheme is based upon the type of examination required for passing the Part II of the MRCOphth (UK) Examination. As with all clinical examination techniques, it is always important to tailor the examination to the individual patient and some of the following steps may not always be necessary. However, by following all of them religiously, many errors in refraction will hopefully be avoided. Well-polished, the following routine can take as little as 15 minutes with a suitable patient.

Entire textbooks are written on the art of refraction. The set of steps below are merely designed as an aide-mémoire and should not be regarded as a substitute for further reading, or preferably spending time with optometrists, who, in the main, are incredibly skilled in the art. Never be ashamed to admit that your efforts at refraction are probably not as polished as a qualified, card-carrying optometrist!

This chapter is designed to be read specifically in conjunction with Chapters 8 ('Retinoscopy'), 9 ('Maddox rod') and 10 ('Cross-cylinders'). Furthermore, it is recommended that the reader has assimilated the rest of the 'Basic clinical optics' section prior to attempting to read this chapter for the first time.

Suggested scheme for Examinations

- Introduce oneself to the patient, followed by a relevant preamble.
- Take a brief relevant history:
  - name and age
  - ocular history, including medications (especially miotics and mydriatics)
  - diabetes mellitus
  - other medical history and medications
  - occupation, e.g. jeweller, watch-maker (specialised needs)
  - hobbies, e.g. sewing, reading, other hobbies requiring near vision
  - any other special reading requirements
  - computer use (may require intermediate correction).
- Test the visual acuity:
  - distance vision (with the lights on), unaided, with spectacles (if allowed) and with pinhole (if vision worse than 6/6).
  - near vision (in a good light) without spectacles (and with reading spectacles if allowed). At this stage, an important clue regarding the patient's refraction can be

gained if they are myopic: the unaided reading vision will be excellent compared to the unaided distance vision. In addition, the degree of myopia can be assessed by the distance that the patient chooses to hold the near test plates from the eyes.

- Perform a cover test (see 'Cover testing', Ch. 29) for distance (using the lowest letter on the chart visible with either eye, or light if no letters visible) and for near. Manifest strabismus in the absence of diplopia may make any future binocular tests irrelevant.

- Measure the interpupillary distance (IPD) in millimetres: e.g. 'Look into my left eye', while placing ruler over temporal limbus of patient's right eye, then 'Look into my right eye', noting the reading on the ruler of the patient's nasal limbus of the left eye.

- Set the trial frame to the IPD and place carefully onto patient's face.

- Dim the lights for the first time. Ask the patient to stare at either the red light of the duochrome or the white spot of the light box (both are acceptable).

- Make quick passes with the retinoscope in both eyes (see 'Retinoscopy', Ch. 8). Ensure that both eyes are fogged (i.e. not accommodating): there should be an *against* movement in all meridia in both eyes at your chosen working distance with the retinoscope cuff down—if not, add more '+' lenses to the trial frame and retinoscope again.

- Check your working distance (usually 66 cm or 50 cm, mostly dependent on personal preference and the length of your arms). Ensure that you are at the same height as the patient and are not 'off-axis'; if so, errors will be generated, particularly with cylindrical corrections.

- Ensure that during retinoscopy your head does not obstruct the patient's line of vision; this can lead to accommodation and therefore spurious results.

- Retinoscope the right eye, if possible using dynamic techniques (i.e. moving towards and away from the patient while performing retinoscopy; see box below). If no clear reflex is seen with initial retinoscopy passes, try adding high '+' or '−' lenses and repeating the manoeuvre.

Further Information

Dynamic techniques in retinoscopy

For each meridian, the reciprocal of the (new) working distance in metres (i.e. the distance from the patient at the point of neutralisation), when subtracted from the total sphere in the trial frame, is the approximate refraction for that meridian. For example, if neutralisation is seen in the 090 meridian at 20 cm from the patient, and there is a +2 D sphere in the trial frame (and the patient was fogged prior to dynamic manoeuvres), then the likely refraction for this meridian is approximately −3 D (2 − (1/0.2)).

Although this sounds frighteningly advanced, try it with a high myope and no lenses in the trial frame (auto-fogged!): e.g. a −10 D myope will neutralise at approximately 10 cm from the eye. Then try inserting −8.5 D and repeating retinoscopy at a normal working distance of 66 cm (equivalent to +1.5 D) to fine tune the refraction: it looks very impressive, *if you know what you are doing.*

Basic clinical optics

- Then retinoscope the left eye.
- Put the room lights on.
- Write down the retinoscopy result (either prescription or power cross).
- Write down your working distance at conclusion of retinoscopy. Remove the appropriate amount of sphere from the trial frame for your working distance, e.g. remove 1.5 D if final working distance is 66 cm, or 2 D for 50 cm.
- Occlude the left eye and test the new right visual acuity. Then occlude the right eye and test the left visual acuity.
- Occlude the left eye (unless asked to perform binocular refraction, in which case fog the left eye instead with +1 D, which should reduce visual acuity to < 6/18; ensure that this is the case).
- Ask the patient to look at the line above the lowest line that they can read clearly. Add +0.5 D to the right eye asking, 'does that make it any worse?' Continue adding '+' sphere until it is worse. Then try ± 0.25 or 0.5 D, asking the patient if they prefer lens '1 or 2'. Ensure that 'better' is not the same as 'smaller and blacker'.
- Now check the cylinder with cross-cylinders (Ch. 10). Ask the patient to stare at a letter 'O' on the chart that they can see clearly (e.g. 6/24 level). Ask which position of the cross-cylinder makes it look rounder (axis), then adjust the axis according to the patient's preference. Then, to test the power of the cylinder, ask the patient which orientation of the cross-cylinder makes the 'O' look sharper. If there appear to be odd replies with testing the axis, check the power of the cylinder—there may be no cylinder to speak of. Similar errors arise when one assumes that the colour red on a cross-cylinder always implies positive cylinder—it is not always so.
- While adjusting the power of the cylinder, adjust the sphere if appropriate. For example, if the patient prefers an additional +0.5 D cylinder in a particular meridian, remember that, when added, such a cylinder will also have a positive spherical equivalent of half this value, i.e. +0.25 D. Therefore, before retesting the patient's vision with the new cylinder, subtract 0.25 D from the spherical slot of the trial frame.
- When finished with the cylinder, recheck the sphere firstly by trying to add more '+' lenses. Then ask if the patient prefers ±0.25 D lenses. Again, ensure that 'better' is not the same as 'smaller and blacker'. Remember that although the patient may be able to read the lowest line on the chart while wearing many different corrections, you have only done a good refraction if the prescription is the least *minus* (or most positive); therefore encourage as much '+' as possible, provided visual acuity does not suffer.
- Record the new visual acuity.
- Repeat for the other eye. Record the visual acuity.
- Record the binocular visual acuity. Try adding binocular +0.25 D (especially in the young) and see if it is well tolerated; if so, try adding more.
- In order to try and eliminate accommodation, use the duochrome bar for each eye in turn. Ideally, the black letters should be seen clearer on the red background than on the green; if not, try adding small amounts of '+' lenses to make this so before rechecking visual acuity, which should not fall.

This step is often excluded in pseudophakes, as there should be no accommodation.

- Dim the lights again. Place a Maddox rod (Ch. 9) in front of the right eye and ask the patient to stare at the white dot on the light box. If required, add prisms to the right eye to bring the red line (of the Maddox rod) to meet the white dot in both the vertical and horizontal meridia.

- Turn the lights on again in order to test near vision. Provide extra lights if at all possible. Bearing the age of the patient in mind, test near vision with a test-type chart/book, adding equal reading 'adds' to both eyes if required. Remember that for a pseudophakic patient, +3 D often works very adequately. In an Examination situation, it is wise to spend a little while obviously counselling the patient about whether this is the 'right distance for you?…what about computing?… and what about for your interest in philately?… etc.'

 Highlight

Suggested reading 'adds'

Age 45–50: 0–1 D; 50–55yrs: 1–1.75 D; 55–60yrs: 1.5–2.25 D; 60+: 1.75–2.5 D

Add = Patient's dioptric normal reading distance $- \frac{1}{2} \times$ (amplitude of residual accommodation (D)), where the dioptric reading distance is the reciprocal of the reading distance in metres (e.g. 3 D if reading distance is 33 cm (0.33 m)).

- Record the near visual acuity.
- Measure back vertex distance—if applicable (generally for prescriptions over 5 D, but good practice to measure it in everybody if preparing for exams; you will forget otherwise!).
- In an examination, it is sometimes necessary to measure a near phoria, which can be done using the Maddox wing. This is a rather old piece of equipment, which often produces spurious results and is not dealt with further here.
- Construct the overall prescription, transposing it if necessary.
- When finished, remove the trial frame, replace the lenses carefully and thank the patient.

Section 2
Ophthalmic equipment

Technical use of the slitlamp

SN Madge

Introduction

Appropriate use of the slitlamp is a vital skill for the trainee ophthalmologist. It is the single most used piece of equipment in the clinic setting, allowing high magnification of ocular structures and practical procedures (such as the removal of corneal foreign bodies) to be performed. As a binocular instrument, it allows a stereoscopic view of the eye, so revealing detail that is impossible to appreciate with monocular equipment, such as the direct ophthalmoscope. In addition, it may be used with appropriate lenses (see below) to view the fundus.

This chapter is essentially concerned with the technical aspects of the machine, its settings and controls; for its use in clinical examination of the eye, please refer to Chapter 32 ('Examination of the anterior segment with the slitlamp') and Chapter 33 ('Retinal examination at the slitlamp').

Basic principles

The slitlamp is a binocular compound microscope, which in optical terms is relatively low powered. Its working distance, the distance between the distal lens and the subject, is quite long, which allows instrumentation on the cornea (or in the anterior chamber) to be possible. The slitlamp has a rotating illumination arm, which, unless uncoupled from the microscope, maintains a direct illumination of the area in focus through the eye-pieces (confocality).

Each eyepiece arm of the microscope contains two convex lenses, which form inverted, virtual images of the eye. The two images are then laterally and vertically inverted through the use of two Porro prisms, so finally producing erect, but virtual images. The two eyepiece arms are inclined at approximately 13° to each other, allowing comfortable binocular viewing.

Controls

There are many makes and types of slitlamp, so it is important to familiarise yourself with the controls of each machine.

- Standard tabletop mounted machines should have a switch just under the tabletop to turn the lamp on, usually with three or more power settings. A lever for adjusting the height of the machine is also usually found under the tabletop.

- Look at the eyepieces and ensure that they are fully pushed into the slitlamp (Fig. 12.1). Under standard use, the eyepieces produce × 10 magnification, but

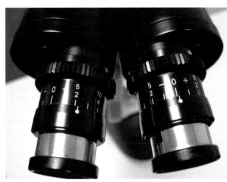

Fig. 12.1 Slitlamp eyepieces. Check the eyepieces are fully pushed in before use. Also ensure that the ± dial reads approximately zero, unless you wish to dial in your own refractive correction and not wear spectacles.

if required, these eyepieces can be pulled from their sockets and replaced with × 16 equivalents, which are often housed in a drawer on the undersurface or side of the lamp. Unless you wear spectacles and prefer to remove them for work, ensure that the dial on each eyepiece reads approximately zero (some people routinely choose –1 or –2 D for each eye, due to the convergence and accommodation that the converging eyepiece arms induce).

- Part the eyepieces to match your interpupillary distance—a single image will be visible through the eyepieces when both are used simultaneously.

- Immediately below the eyepieces is often a magnification lever, with low power to the left and high power to the right. More advanced machines may instead incorporate whole banks of Galilean telescopes for higher powered viewing, which are operated by rotating the desired power lens into position (these lens banks are located in the main body of the slitlamp microscope and not under the eyepieces).

- The slitlamp's base is quite mobile on the tabletop, provided that its brake is off—unscrew anticlockwise to allow movement and replace the brake if the table itself is to be moved; this will help to prevent damage to the lamp.

- The machine's base can be pushed around the tabletop with relatively gross movements, but finer control is possible through use of the joystick. In addition to movements in the plane of the table, rotating the joystick will lead to vertical movements of the lamp.

- The illumination column is quite complex:

  - At the very top lies the bulb, which may be changed by unscrewing or unclipping its cover (ensure that electrical power is switched off). Beware the bulb can be very hot if in recent use!

  - Below the bulb cover is a dial, which may be adjusted by the screw knob (A) below (Fig. 12.2). This dial allows changes between blue light (used to fluoresce the chemical dye fluorescein), a slit of white light (in gradations of millimetres of height) and usually a spot of light.

  - Between the knob and the dial is a switch (B) which controls the type of light produced by the slitlamp. From left to right, these settings produce unfiltered light (which should never be used to examine the retina), heat-filtered light, neutral density-filtered light (less bright), red-free light (used to examine the vitreous body and retinal vessels) and an empty slot for additional filters as required.

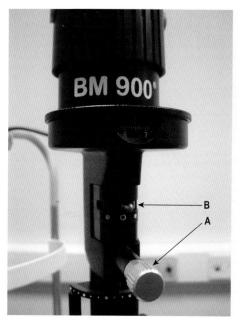

Fig. 12.2 Illumination column. Knob (A) allows changes between the cobalt blue filtered light (used to excite fluorescein) and the slit beam, whose height is also adjusted by turning the knob. Switch (B) controls the type of light produced by the slitlamp, changing between unfiltered light, heat-filtered light, neutral density-filtered light (less bright), red-free light (green) and often an empty slot.

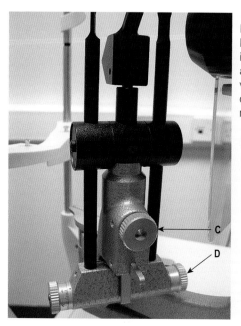

Fig. 12.3 Illumination column. Turning knob (C) anticlockwise uncouples the illumination column from the microscope, allowing illumination of one structure while viewing another. Dial (D) controls the width of the slit beam; it is calibrated in millimetres.

- The illumination column may be rotated to lie coaxial with the microscope or to one side of it, so changing the type of illumination of the eye.

- In addition to lateral movement, the light source may be rotated in the vertical plane by carefully unclipping the bottom of the column and rotating it forward or backward as required.

- The illumination column can be partially uncoupled from the microscope by turning screw C (Fig. 12.3); this allows illumination of one structure while viewing another, as in the technique of sclerotic scatter (light passes from the illuminated limbus through the cornea by total internal reflection, making corneal opacities readily visible; see Ch. 32).

- On either side of the bottom of the illumination column lies another dial (D), again calibrated in millimetres (Fig. 12.3). This dial controls the width of the slit beam, often doubling as a 'stand by' switch, if the lamp is to be turned off temporarily.

- Further screws at the junction of the microscope and the illumination column can be tightened to immobilise the slit lamp on the illumination column or base, or a combination thereof.

- The patient should be positioned on the head rest so that the eyes lie in line with the black line on the lateral supporting columns. If this is not the case, the height of the face can be adjusted with a dial on the side of the patient support, but it is important to avoid hurting the patient in such a manoeuvre. In addition, consider whether vertical movements of the entire slit lamp and table might be useful in making the patient more comfortable.

- Also found on the side of the patient's head rest is a small light which can occasionally be a useful fixation target.

13

Indirect ophthalmoscopy and scleral indentation

SN Madge

Introduction

Indirect ophthalmoscopes vary in design, style and age, but the basic principles remain the same. In Royal College Examinations, one can generally expect to be offered the more old-fashioned types of equipment to use and it is therefore very worthwhile ensuring that you have had experience with all common types.

The main advantages of the indirect ophthalmoscope over slitlamp examination are:

- portability
- wider field of view
- brighter light source for examination through media opacities
- the possibility of dynamic vitreoretinal examination using scleral indentation
- the ability (if required) to adapt the headset to incorporate a laser for retinal treatment, which is of great value for treatment under general anaesthesia.

Furthermore, a teaching mirror can be fitted to the front of the headset to allow an observer to gain a similar image (albeit not of the same quality) to the examiner.

Principles

A convex lens (known as a condensing lens and typically a +20 D) is held in front of the patient's eye as the light source (from the headset) is shone through it. Light reflected from the retina is focused by the condensing lens to a point between the examiner and the lens, forming an optically real image of the retina (Fig. 13.1).

The eyepieces of the ophthalmoscope usually contain +2 D lenses, allowing relaxation of accommodation and thus easy viewing of the image at arm's length even in presbyopia (arm's length is approximately 50 cm, explaining the choice of +2 D lenses). The image is inverted (as per slitlamp examination with +90 D lens) and varies in its size and field of view dependent on the refractive error of the patient (see below), the pupil sizes of both the patient and examiner, and the power of the condensing lens.

A higher power lens (e.g. 30 D) will produce a smaller image but a larger field of view.

Ophthalmic equipment

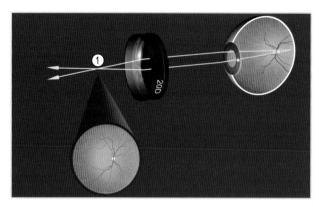

Fig 13.1 Indirect ophthalmoscopy. This diagram shows the subject's eye and the condensing lens. The observer is to the left of the diagram. During indirect ophthalmoscopy, it is recommended that the condensing lens be kept perpendicular to the observer's visual axis at all times. The real, inverted image is formed between the observer and the condensing lens (1).

How to do it

Most trainees can be taught to use the indirect within a few minutes; however, learning to use it well can take many months.

- After putting on the headset, adjust the various knobs until a steady fit is achieved, and turn the power on. Next, look through each eyepiece in turn, ensuring that the image seen is centred and that the same image is seen through either eye; the eyepieces are adjustable and will move horizontally to accommodate large and small interpupillary distances (Fig. 13.2). If the light spot seen is vertically displaced, then it can be brought to the correct level by altering the tilt of the mirror on the headset (often using a lever on the side).

- Look with both eyes together at a target approximately 50 cm away (e.g. one's thumb) and ensure that only one image is appreciated. If you are having trouble (and are possibly diplopic!), it may be that your indirect has a further control for adjusting the distance between the prismatic eyepieces (can enhance stereopsis)—adjust according to comfort and your horizontal fusion range. Unless you are hypermetropic, you will soon realise that distant objects are out of focus when seen through the eyepieces—this is, of course, due to the incorporated +2 D lenses. Significantly ametropic examiners should leave their spectacles on while examining with the indirect ophthalmoscope, or use a bespoke indirect ophthalmoscope.

- Paramount to success in examining patients (and also in Examinations) is the comfort of the patient. Indirect ophthalmoscopy in adults is best done with the patient recumbent on an examination couch, allowing plenty of access for the examiner to move around the couch where necessary.

- Ensure that the room lights are dimmed and that the patient has a well-dilated pupil (if the pupil is small, consider using a smaller spot size—a switch on the headset should oblige).

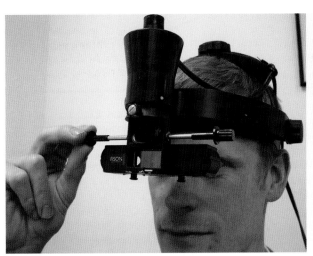

Fig 13.2 Adjusting the indirect ophthalmoscope headset. The eyepieces may be adjusted horizontally to accommodate different interpupillary distances. The vertical displacement of the light spot can also be adjusted.

- In formal examinations, it is wise to start by examining the retinal periphery so as not to startle the patient with a bright light in the central vision (!). For beginners, it is recommended that a low light source be used, and that one concentrates on looking at the posterior pole (e.g. ask the patient to look at your ear—right ear for right eye, left ear for left eye).

- Grasp the lens between thumb and forefinger, resting at least one of your remaining fingers on the patient's forehead to steady yourself. Ensure that you are holding the lens at arm's length, while making sure that it remains perpendicular to the axis between your headset and the patient's eyes. If one side of the lens is coloured white (on its rim), then place this side closest to the patient; this provides the least optical aberrations if using an aspheric lens.

- With the lens practically touching the patient, shine the light through the lens. There should be an obvious, non-inverted but magnified view of the pupil, iris and anterior segment. Keeping these structures in view, and ensuring that the lens remains perpendicular to the axis at all times, gently move the lens towards you. After only a few centimetres, the blackness of the enlarging pupil will suddenly change into the orange glow of the retina.

- Focus this now inverted image by moving the lens back and forth. If the image is lost, simply push the lens back towards the pupil until the anterior segment becomes visible and, keeping the lens perpendicular, pull away slowly again.

- To examine more peripheral areas, ask the patient to look in the desired direction (e.g. 'look up' to examine the superior retina) and remember to keep the lens perpendicular to the axis. Traditionally (and certainly in the Examination setting), it is best to move around the patient examining, for example, the temporal retina of the right eye from the left side of the patient, and the inferior retina from a standing position above the head.

Troubleshooting

- If you are struggling to get an image, or find that your image quality is poor, it is probably due to one of two reasons:

  1. Excessive movement of the lens. Ensure that your remaining fingers are firmly on the patient's forehead. If the problem persists, try a two-handed approach.

  2. Your lens is not perpendicular to the axis between your headset and the patient's eye. Bring the lens back towards the eye and start again, concentrating on not tilting the lens as you bring it back towards yourself.

- 'There isn't a round spot of light coming out of the headset—just an image of the bulb…' This is normal for older-style equipment and will provide as good an image as the newer-style indirect ophthalmoscopes.

Other lenses

A +28 D (or +30 D) lens is very useful for examining the retinal periphery, as it gives a wider field of view, albeit with lower magnification. It is therefore the lens of choice in paediatric ophthalmology, in particular the screening of possible cases of retinopathy of prematurity. This lens is also invaluable for vitreoretinal specialists, as it facilitates a far better retinal image in the presence of intra-ocular gas than is possible with the +20 D lens.

A +13 D lens can also be useful to gain a magnified view of the optic disc and is sometimes used in paediatric ophthalmology.

Ametropia

Moving the lens away from a myopic eye will cause the image seen to increase in size, whereas the converse is true in hypermetropia.

Scleral indentation

Indentation is a technique used to obtain views of the retinal periphery and ora serrata, which also gives information on the dynamic vitreoretinal interface (e.g. retinal tears with ongoing vitreoretinal traction). Examination should always be from the opposite side of the patient and it is important to move around the patient to obtain the best views.

- It is recommended that topical anaesthetic be instilled in both eyes prior to the procedure (allows prolonged fixation and reduced conjunctival sensation in temporal and nasal retinal examination). Warn the patient that, despite the anaesthetic, the examination is likely to be slightly uncomfortable, but should not be painful.

- Stand above the patient's head and ask the patient to look at you. Place the indenter in the lower lid crease and then ask the patient to look down (Fig. 13.3).

- Obtain a view of the inferior peripheral retina in the manner described above.

- Apply gentle pressure perpendicular to the globe in the region of the ora serrata, while watching the lower part of the image: the dynamic indent should appear. Do not push posteriorly as this will cause pain.

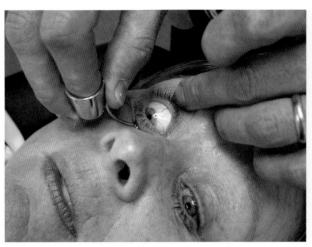

Fig. 13.3 Scleral indentation. First ask the patient to look up towards you. Place the indenter in the lower lid crease and then ask the patient to look down (i.e. in the direction of the indenter).

- If no image appears, try looking a little more peripherally; do not push harder.
- It is recommended that, when learning the technique of indentation, patients with larger than average orbits are selected first. Patients with small, deep-set eyes are often very difficult to examine and it is easy to hurt them.

Troubleshooting

- *'I hurt my patients.'* You are probably pushing posteriorly too much and possibly too hard. Try angling the gentle pressure applied into the globe itself, not posteriorly into the orbit.
- *'I can't see the indent.'* You are either:
  (i) not looking peripherally enough
  (ii) not looking at the same part of the eye that you are indenting—check by moving the lens out of the way temporarily
  (iii) indenting either too anteriorly or too posteriorly—think about the surface landmarks of the ora serrata and peripheral retina
  (iv) in need of more practice with the indirect alone.

Indirect laser

The combination of an indirect-mounted laser and scleral indentation allows even the most peripherally located retinal lesions to be dealt with. Laser spot size is often a little unpredictable, making this technique unsafe for macular laser treatments. Functions such as laser power, duration and 'repeat' are all applicable to the indirect laser as well. For more information on the use of the argon laser, see Chapter 49 ('Ophthalmic therapeutic lasers').

In general, the condensing lens is held still while the laser is moved around by small movements of the examiner's head. It is suggested that, in order to minimise the risk from a stray laser shot, the other eye is covered during the procedure.

Direct ophthalmoscopy

SN Madge

Introduction

The direct ophthalmoscope is usually only occasionally used by ophthalmologists, but does provide excellent magnified views of the posterior segment, albeit with a grossly reduced field of view. It is therefore useful for examining the optic disc for haemorrhages (especially in glaucoma) and retinal vein pulsation. From an Examination point of view, it is vital to be au fait with its use. This chapter will provide a general schema which should be acceptable in such situations.

Principles

The direct ophthalmoscope emits a diverging beam of light into the patient's eye, which illuminates the retina, reflecting light back towards the observer. An erect, virtual image of the retina is seen, which, dependent on the refractive state of both observer and patient, may require focusing—either by accommodation or using the built-in focusing lenses of the ophthalmoscope.

The field of view and magnification are highly dependent on the refractive state of the patient, with myopes providing a greater degree of magnification and smaller field of view than emmetropic patients. The converse is true in hypermetropia. The field of view is greater in patients with widely dilated pupils and also increases with increasing proximity to the patient.

The anterior segment of the eye can also be examined with the direct ophthalmoscope by using the built-in lenses and light as a self-illuminating loupe (magnifying glass). By increasing the lens power to ≈+15–20 D and observing the patient from ≈5 cm distance, a magnified view of these structures can be appreciated.

As the images involved are virtual, the optics of the situation mean that patient movement is grossly amplified. This means that small amounts of nystagmus can be easily picked up; however, with larger and more rapid excursions, indirect ophthalmoscopy may provide a better way of imaging the fundus.

The equipment

Most ophthalmoscopes have a variable spot size (smaller better for small pupils) and a red filter (green light) for examining retinal vasculature. All should have a focusing wheel, usually bringing *plus* (usually black coloured) lenses into action with clockwise rotation, and *minus* lenses (usually red coloured) with anticlockwise rotation. Other features may include fixation crosses and a blue filter for use with fluorescein.

How to do it

The following schema provides a comprehensive checklist ideal for Examinations.

- Introduction to the patient. Turn down the room lights.
- Ask the patient to fixate a particular object in the distance (e.g. light switch, coat hook, etc.). Tell the patient to relax and 'remember to keep breathing'—many will attempt to breath hold otherwise, which will cause a degree of anxiety.
- Use your right hand and eye for the patient's right eye and vice versa.
- Using a broad spot light from the distance, compare the pupil sizes and if not dilated, consider checking for a relative afferent pupillary defect (RAPD). (Direct ophthalmoscopy in Examinations often feature patients with optic nerve pathology, when an RAPD would certainly be useful information.) See Chapter 28 ('Examination of the pupils') for more information.
- Examine the anterior segment (using a +15–20 D lens) unless told not to.
- Again from a distance, check the red reflexes (Fig. 14.1). Are there lens opacities present?
- Place your non-examining hand on the patient (explaining to the patient that you are steadying yourself), either on the shoulder or forehead above the eye in question (Fig. 14.2). This is an important manoeuvre to do, as it will be very difficult to maintain a steady view without some form of 'anchor'.
- Reduce the spot size of the ophthalmoscope if the pupils are very miosed.

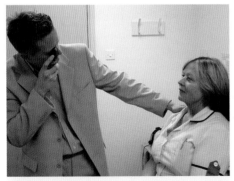

Fig 14.1 Checking red reflexes. Before approaching the patient, check the patient's red reflexes from a distance.

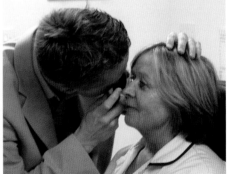

Fig. 14.2 Getting a steady view. In order to get a steady view, it is recommended that you gently hold on to the patient. However, it is important to tell the patient what you are doing!

- Move slowly towards the patient, keeping the red reflex in view, approaching from temporal to and just above the patient's line of fixation. Examine the posterior pole of the eye, starting with the disc. Rotate the focusing dial if necessary to obtain a clear view—remember to use the least amount of *minus* lenses necessary, otherwise your accommodation will be stimulated (see below). Get as close to the patient as possible without touching.

- Examine the disc's colour, cup and contours. From the disc, follow the vascular arcades towards the periphery, noting any arteriovenous nipping, sheathing, etc. Repeat this for all the different arcades.

- Examine the peripheral retina by asking the patient to look in the direction of interest.

- Finally, ask the patient to look at the light; this will hopefully bring the macula into view.

- If relevant, consider using the red filter (green light) at this stage; this should highlight vascular anomalies.

- Make a mental note of the number on the lens dial; this will provide a clue to the approximate refractive correction of the patient's eye (see below).

- Repeat for the other eye.

Troubleshooting

- *'Should I leave my spectacles on?'* The ophthalmoscope can only correct for spherical errors, so if you have a significant amount of astigmatism, it may be better to leave your spectacles on. However, most people remove their spectacles and dial their spherical prescription into the ophthalmoscope (e.g. a −4 D myope would dial in 'red' −4).

- *'Should I leave the patient's spectacles on?'* In most cases it is better to remove them, except in the case of high myopes, where the view is usually better with the spectacles in place.

- *'How do I work out the patient's approximate refractive prescription?'* The key to understanding this is to appreciate that, as the images involved are virtual, the rays forming a perfectly focused image are in fact parallel, not focused to a point. The patient's prescription is roughly the number on the dial of the ophthalmoscope, corrected for your own prescription, provided that you (and the patient!) are not accommodating. These approximations become less accurate with higher refractive errors.

    - To reduce the amount of accommodation exerted by yourself, once you have a clear view, rotate the dial slowly clockwise until the image starts to become blurred. In this way, you will be tolerating the most amount of *plus* lens possible, thus dampening accommodation.

    - To prevent the patient accommodating, ask the patient to maintain a steady distance fixation.

    - *'Give me an example.'* You are a −2 D myope examining a patient with both your and the patient's spectacles off. You are able to get a clear image with the number +4 dialled into the ophthalmoscope, and the addition of more *plus* lenses (clockwise rotation) makes the image blurred. Your 2 D of myopia (meaning that your eye is too powerful) are helping to refract the otherwise diverging rays from the patient (and make them more parallel) and are therefore effectively functioning as an extra +2 D lens. Thus, the patient's prescription is approximately (+4) + (+2) = +6 D hypermetropic.

- *'And another.'* You are a −3 D myope examining a patient with both your and the patient's spectacles off. You notice that you can get an equally clear image of the patient's disc with numbers on the dial between −6 and −9 D. Disregard the most *minus* lenses, as these lenses will have been stimulating your accommodation, leaving a lens of −6 D. In order for a clear image to be seen, the ophthalmoscope lenses will need to correct for your −3 D myopia as well, thus only leaving −3 D attributable to the patient.

- *'The patient's optic disc looks oval—why?'* Marked astigmatism may be responsible.

- *'I can see the retina but can't find the disc!'* With practice, it is easy to approach the patient and land on the disc every time. If you are struggling, try following the vessels 'upstream' by observing in which direction they are dividing. All vessels, of course, originate at the disc.

Using the focimeter

MJ Hawker

Introduction

The focimeter is used to measure the power of a spherical lens, the axes and powers of an astigmatic lens and the power of a prism. It is an essential piece of equipment to be able to use, not only for examination purposes but also to enable refractive planning in cataract surgery. There are different designs of focimeter, each with varying modes of operation. However, the principles of use are the same for each. It is recommended that this chapter be read in conjunction with the 'Basic clinical optics' section. As in many areas of ophthalmology, the manual focimeter is being increasingly replaced by an automated variant; however, Examination candidates are unlikely to have the liberty of using such equipment!

Principles

Focimeters allow the measurement of the power of lenses. They consist of a focusing system, which produces the image viewed by an observation system (viewing telescope). Diverging light from a source passes through a card with a ring of holes in it, and then to a collimating lens (which converges light rays to make them parallel and therefore produces a focused image of a ring of dots). If the lens to be tested is placed between the collimating lens and the viewing telescope, the light will be refracted by the test lens and the image viewed will be blurred. By adjusting the distance of the card from the collimating lens, the light reaching the collimating lens can be made more or less divergent. If this adjustment is equal and opposite to the effect of the test lens, a focused image is produced and the power can be read off a calibrated scale.

How to do it

- Turn on the machine.
- Before testing, set the instrument to zero, turn the eyepiece fully anticlockwise, then clockwise until the dots and the graticule have just come into focus (this ensures you are not accommodating to focus the image).
- Place the patient's spectacles on the rest in the upright position and with the spectacle arms at the back (the posterior surface of the lens is then in contact with the lens rest, in order to measure the *back vertex power*) (Fig. 15.1). Each lens is measured in turn, conventionally starting with the right lens.

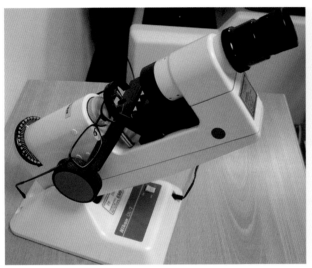

Fig. 15.1 Focimeter placement. Place the spectacles on the focimeter in the upright position with the spectacle arms at the back.

- Adjust the position of the spectacle lens to place the image (ring of dots) in the centre of the graticule. This locates the lens optical centre. If the image cannot be centred, a prismatic element is present.

- A sharp ring of dots is seen if: (i) only a sphere is present and (ii) the collimating lens is focused. If the dots are drawn out, a cylindrical element is present.

- Adjust the instrument using the focusing wheel (power drum) until the image is focused. Read the power in dioptres from the numerical scale, noting whether the power is positive or negative. If the lens is spherical, this is the only reading required.

- If a cylinder is present, the dots form lines. These are: (i) focused by adjusting the focusing wheel and (ii) made linear (and less blurred) by turning the cylinder axis wheel. The adjustment of the axis is crucial to obtaining a focused image, and even more so with higher powered cylindrical elements. Record the power in dioptres (this is the sphere power). Note that stronger cylinders cast longer lines.

- Further adjust the focusing wheel so that the image lines become refocused at 90° to the first image. The power of the cylinder is equal to the difference between the first and second power readings. Record the axis of the cylinder by observing the direction of the lines of the second image. Some instruments have a graticule in the eyepiece that can be rotated to align with the lines of the image and record the axis.

- As an example, consider the examination of a lens on the focimeter of prescription +3.00/−4.75 × 045 (Fig. 15.2). With the spectacles placed on the machine, the power drum is turned until the lines cast by the lens are found to be focused at +3.00 D, the lines pointing at 135 degrees. As the drum is turned down, the second image becomes focused at −1.75 D, with the lines pointing at 045 degrees. The difference in the two readings represents the

Ophthalmic equipment

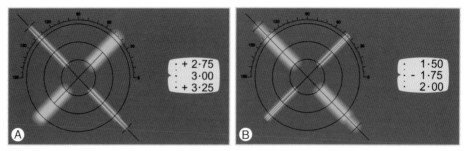

Fig. 15.2 Example of lens examination using a modern focimeter, which produces an image of a cross rather than dots. A. The lines that are in focus indicate that the lens has a power of +3.00 D with an axis of 135°. **B.** The lines that are now in focus indicate that the lens also has a power of −1.75 D with an axis of 45°.

amount of astigmatism present, i.e. 4.75 D (+3.00 − (−1.75) = 4.75). The prescription is thus either +3.00/−4.75 × 045 (in *minus* cylinder notation) or −1.75/+4.75 × 135 (*plus* cylinder). Note that the reading given by the focimeter is not a power reading, but an axis reading (power of cylinder is at 90° to the axis), with the focimeter providing the axis of the cylinder as it appears in the prescription.

- Depending on which of the two images cast by a spherocylindrical lens is viewed first, either a negative or a positive cylinder will be recorded.

Bifocals

- If the spectacles contain bifocal lenses, the strength of the *add* is calculated by the difference in power between the distance and near segments. For small amounts of *add*, it is acceptable to calculate this from the back vertex powers. However, for stronger *add*, the difference in front vertex powers should be used (by placing the lens with its front surface against the lens rest).

- If it is not possible to centre the image, a prismatic element is present. Note that on the focimeter, the image is deviated towards the base of the prism— the opposite of when looking through a prism where the image is deviated towards the prism apex (see 'Basic clinical optics' section). This is because the image is inverted by the eyepiece telescope on the focimeter.

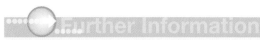

Further Information

Measuring prismatic elements using the focimeter

If a prism is incorporated into the prescription, it will not be possible to centre the image on the focimeter graticule. Prisms that are incorporated into spectacles have an equivalent effect relative to each eye. Therefore, a 2 D base-up prism in the right lens has an equivalent effect to a 2 D base-down prism in the left lens. Similarly, a 2 D base-out prism in the right lens has an equivalent effect to a 2 D base-out prism in the left lens. The effect is additive between the two eyes. Therefore, 3 D base-up and 3 D base-in in the left lens, with 3 D base-down and 3 D base-in in the right is equivalent to 6 D base-up and 6 D base-in in the left alone, or 6 D base-down and 6 D base-in in the right alone.

The focimeter graticule has a series of concentric rings (or marks, depending on the make) of increasing size, orientated about the centre of the scale. The distance between each ring represents 1 dioptre of prism power of deviation of the image away from the centre. When a prism is present, the image on the focimeter is deviated towards the base of the prism in the spectacle lens. Conventionally, prisms in spectacles are described by the direction of their base, and so the focimeter maintains this convention.

To measure the strength and direction of prism incorporated into a prescription:

- Whilst the patient is wearing the spectacles, use a lens marker to mark the position of the centre of each pupil on each lens. This marks the effective optical axis that each eye is using with each lens.
- Place the spectacles on the focimeter. Starting on the right, centre the lens so that the pupil mark lies over the centre of the focimeter stop.
- Adjust the focusing wheel until the image is focused.
- The strength of prism is measured, usually in 1 D increments, by noting the position of the centre of the image relative to the concentric marks on the graticule. If a cylinder is present, the image will be elongated in one meridian. However, it is still the position of the centre of the image that marks the power of the prismatic deviation.
- The direction of the prism is noted by the direction of deviation of the image by the spectacle lens. Thus, for example, upward deviation of the image denotes a base-up prism.
- The process is repeated for the left spectacle lens.
- Note that if a prism has been introduced into the prescription only by decentration of the optical axis of the lens relative to the patient's pupil, and not by additional incorporation of prism, then it will still be possible to centre the image on the focimeter. The prismatic element might then be missed if the operator is not alert to the deviation of the optical centre of the lens away from a position consistent with the patient's pupil.

Keratometry

SN Madge

Introduction

Keratometers provide measurements of the curvature of the cornea. Such measurements are used in ocular biometry and also complement information gleaned from refractive data, which can then be used in planning refractive procedures. As such, it is recommended that this chapter be read in conjunction with the 'Basic clinical optics' section and Chapter 7 ('Biometry').

Many modern keratometers are fully automatic; not only do they sense a curved, reflecting surface (i.e. the cornea), but measurements are provided automatically in a form that can be easily understood. However, older pieces of equipment are still to be found in some departments and especially in Examinations. This chapter will briefly discuss the principles involved before describing the use of one kind of keratometer, the Javal–Schiotz type, which has been most commonly found in Examinations.

Principles

As well as allowing light to pass through it, the anterior surface of the cornea also acts as a convex mirror, reflecting some of the light that is incident upon it to produce an image. Mathematical formulae exist that relate (i) the size of the image seen to (ii) the radius of curvature of the cornea, (iii) the distance of the object (responsible for the image) from the cornea and (iv) the size of the object. If three of these measurements are known, then the fourth can be calculated. In the Javal–Schiotz keratometer, the image size and distance are kept constant, while the object size is varied, allowing measurement of the corneal curvature. From the measured radius of corneal curvature (k reading in mm), one can derive corneal power (in dioptres) by assuming a standard refractive index of the cornea.

Two readings are generally taken during keratometry of the cornea, each perpendicular to the other, along the meridia of maximum and minimum curvature (in regular astigmatism). In Chapter 39 ('Corneal topography') are details on more modern pieces of equipment, which can provide useful information in cases of irregular astigmatism.

How to do it

The Javal–Schiotz keratometer has a similar design to the slitlamp, viz a microscope with a light source. However, instead of a solitary bulb light source, this keratometer has two, each of a different shape and colour (Fig. 16.1), which are known as mires.

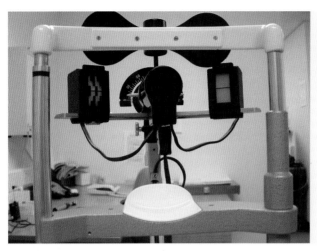

Fig 16.1 The patient's view of the Javal–Schiotz keratometer. Note the two mires of different shapes and colours.

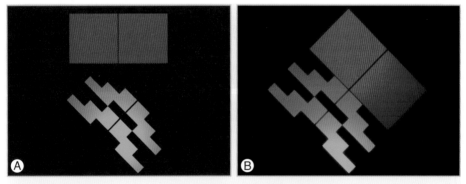

Fig. 16.2 Adjusting difference between mires in keratometry. A. Incorrect position. The mires in this image are aligned to different axes, and there is a significant gap between them. **B.** Correct position. The mires are aligned and (just) touching.

- Ask the patient to move onto the chin rest, and ensure comfort. Make sure that the height is correct and that the forehead meets the headrest. The black marker on the side of the headrest should be level with the eyes.

- Switch on the power. Adjust the eyepiece (to 0 D if emmetropic or spectacles worn) so that the graticule is in focus (occasionally intentionally defocused by examiners!).

- Pull the keratometer back, using the joystick, and roughly align it with one of the patient's eyes. Looking around the side of the machine (not through the eyepieces), check that faint images of the two mires can be made out on the patient's cornea.

- Now look through the eyepiece and bring the reflections on the cornea into focus using the joystick.

- By turning the dial, adjust the distance between the two mires (equivalent to object size) so that the two images are just touching (Fig. 16.2).

- Next rotate the mires so that the central lines, which bisect each of the mires, line-up (Fig. 16.2). It may be necessary to readjust the distance between the mires after rotating them to get an exact reading.

- When the mires are just touching and are perfectly aligned, the keratometry value or *k* reading for that meridian can be read off the scale (in either dioptres or radius of curvature in millimetres).

- Having noted the *k* reading and its meridian, rotate the equipment through 90° and attempt to line up the mires again, adjusting the dials to take the second *k* reading. (NB. Only eyes with regular astigmatism will allow two accurate *k* readings perpendicular to each other.) Note the new reading.

- Repeat for the other eye and ask the patient to sit back.

Troubleshooting

- *'My keratometer is somewhat odd in that it has two dials for meridia, one running from 0 to 180 degrees anticlockwise and another from 0 to 180 degrees clockwise (both on the upper half of the dial). Which do I use?'* The *k* readings are designed to be easily comparable to refractive data. Therefore, use only the dial with 0 to 180 degrees running from right to left, anticlockwise over the top of the dial.

- *'It doesn't matter how much I rotate the dial, the patient's k readings are the same in all meridia.'* Has the patient got a spherical cornea (no astigmatism)?

- *'I can get one reading, but when I rotate the machine through 90 degrees, I cannot get the mires to line up.'* It is certainly possible that your patient has a degree of irregular astigmatism. Consider corneal topography.

- *'The images are moving and my readings don't make sense.'* Ensure that the patient is keeping the head still against the headrest (if not, then the object–cornea distance is varying).

- *'My patient has had refractive surgery previously. Should I flag this up prior to sending the patient to theatre?'* Absolutely. Although you will be able to take keratometry readings from the patient in the usual fashion, it would be invalid to use them in normal biometry calculations in the standard fashion. Consult local protocol to establish what to do.

Gonioscopy and three-mirror examination

SN Madge

Introduction

The smallest of the three mirrors on a Goldmann three-mirror lens can also be used as a gonioscopic lens. The use of these lenses is very similar and thus they are considered together here. In addition, the application to the eye of other contact lenses used for ocular examination (e.g. macular lens) and ophthalmic therapeutic laser is essentially the same as for these lenses.

General principles

The need for the three-mirror and gonioscopic lenses arises as a result of *total internal reflection* of light from peripheral ocular structures. This means that light travelling obliquely from the retinal periphery and anterior drainage angle meets the cornea (specifically the air/cornea interface) and is actually reflected back within the eye, because the angle of incidence of the light exceeds what is known as the *critical angle*. In order to let such light out of the eye (and in order for us to see what is happening in these areas), we must either move the structures to an area where total internal reflection will no longer occur (as in scleral indentation), or alter the cornea/air interface (gonioscopy/three-mirror).

Two main types of gonioscopic lenses exist. All require topical anaesthesia.

- The Goldmann type (gonioscope and three-mirror) is more concave than the cornea and thus a coupling medium (e.g. methylcellulose, some use saline) is required to abolish the air/cornea interface.
- The Zeiss type is less concave than the cornea and can thus be placed directly onto the eye.

In all cases, obliquely travelling light from the ocular peripheries passes through the cornea/lens interface with minimal deviation and then strikes a mirror set within the lens. This reflects the light to the outside of the lens and, as the new direction of travel of the light is practically perpendicular as it crosses the lens/air interface, little or no refraction of light occurs and the peripheral structures are therefore visible.

In the three-mirror lens, each mirror is of a different steepness, allowing views of the post-equatorial, pre-equatorial and ora serrata/drainage angle structures in turn, in addition to the central concave window providing a virtual, erect view of the posterior pole.

Ophthalmic equipment

How to do it

- Set the slitlamp up appropriately (Ch. 32). Most clinicians use the ×16 magnification for gonioscopic evaluation.
- The following routine provides a relatively simple method of getting a lens into position:
  - Allow topical anaesthesia time to work (both eyes).
  - Ensure the patient is at the correct height on the slitlamp chin rest.
  - Ensure that coupling media is applied to the lens, if required.
  - Ask the patient to look down. Lift the upper lid with a finger (Fig 17.1).
  - Ask the patient to look up. Hold the lower lid down with another finger.

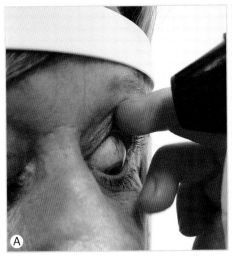

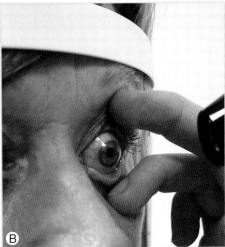

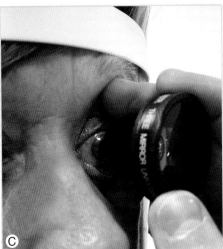

Fig. 17.1 Appling a gonioscopic lens.
To place a contact lens on the cornea, it is often easiest to prevent the lids from blinking the lens away. **A.** Ask the patient to look down and trap the upper lid against the orbital rim. **B.** Ask the patient to look up and then trap the lower lid. **C.** Then place the lens on the cornea.

- With the patient still looking up, and firmly but gently holding the lids, place the lens on the eye, starting with its lower edge and tipping the lens forward under the upper lid. You will need to do this manoeuvre very slickly if using saline as the coupling fluid.

- Politely remind the patient not to move back off the slitlamp and to try (if possible) to refrain from blinking.

- While maintaining a little forward pressure onto the lens, release the lids.

- Focus the slitlamp onto the mirror in question.

- Rotate the lens as required, remembering some forward pressure onto to the lens is necessary to prevent it from coming off.

- Examine the different parts of the eye using the relevant mirror. For gonioscopy, as small a slit as possible is recommended, as light entering the pupil will lead to miosis and possible false interpretation of the angle structures.

- To remove a concave lens when finished, do not simply pull the lens straight off the eye as the induced suction forces may remove all the corneal epithelium too! With the lens still on the eye, apply a little pressure (e.g. with a clean finger) on the globe to the side of the contact lens, which will relieve the suction effect, and/or try gently twisting the lens as you remove it.

Interpretation of angle structures

Interpretation of the structures of the angle is beyond the scope of this book (see Further Reading p. 286). Although pictures of the various types of drainage angles abound, interpretation of gonioscopy in real life can be quite challenging and it is recommended that, for the beginner, a 'tour' of a variety of angles be conducted by a more senior clinician.

Exophthalmometry

JP Kersey

Introduction

This is a method of measuring ocular protrusion. The main difficulty lies in making reproducible measurements. The Hertel exophthalmometer uses a mirror inclined at 45° to the eye to show a side-on view of the anterior segment, while viewing from directly in front of the patient. The main problem is the control of parallax; different exophthalmometers have different methods of managing this, but they all work on the same principle.

How to do it

- The exophthalmometer is adjusted so that the edges of the equipment sit gently on the lateral bony orbital rim (Fig. 18.1).
- Close one of your eyes (in this example, your left). Ask the patient to look at your open eye, for example, if you are measuring the patient's left eye, the patient would be looking at your open right eye.
- Line up the mark on the front of the exophthalmometer (Fig. 18.2, in this case a blue cone) with the middle of the ruler on the mirror (downward mark). You should be able to see a reflection of the corneal apex against the ruler.
- Read off the degree of ocular protrusion in millimetres.
- The process is repeated for the other eye, i.e. measuring the patient's right eye, with your left eye open and your right eye closed.
- When recording the result, it is important to record the distance between the lateral canthi (on the ruler centrepiece of the exophthalmometer) and of course the amount of protrusion for each eye. Measurement of the distance between the lateral canthi allows a more objective comparison to be made between readings (and with time).

Normal measurements are less than 21 mm. Proptosis is defined as a measurement of 22 mm or greater, or a difference of 2 mm between the eyes.

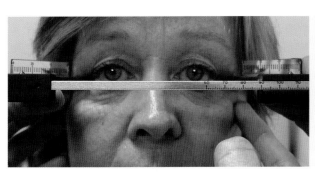

Fig. 18.1 Placing the exophthalmometer. Position yourself level with the patient and carefully place the exophthalmometer on the lateral orbital rims.

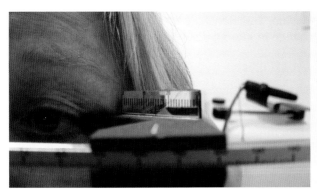

Fig. 18.2 Reading the exophthalmometer. To reduce parallax errors, line up the mark on the front of the exophthalmometer (blue cone here) with the central mark on the millimeter rule (vertical black line in this case).

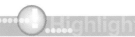 Highlight

Tips and pitfalls

- It is important to repeat measurements with the same intercanthal distance.
- It is important to only use one eye when reading the measurement (avoids parallax).
- Exophthalmos is generally defined as proptosis caused by thyroid eye disease.

Amsler grid testing

MJ Hawker

Introduction

Amsler grid testing (Marc Amsler, Swiss ophthalmologist, 1891–1968) is a quick, useful way of evaluating macular function. The test can be used to screen for disorders or to detect any change in known disease.

Principles

An Amsler chart consists of a 10 cm square grid subdivided into smaller squares. When held 33 cm from the eye, the chart is projected onto the macular area subtending 20° vertically and horizontally (10° in each direction from fixation—normally the foveola). The position of aberrations in the chart perceived by the patient (while fixating the central dot) guides the examiner in looking for anatomical correlates on macular fundoscopy.

In total there are seven different Amsler charts available. Figure 19.1 shows the first in the series, which is divided into 400 smaller 5 mm squares. When viewed at 33 cm, each small square subtends an angle of 1°. Amsler chart 2 is similar to chart 1, but has two diagonal lines from the corners crossing at the central dot. These lines aid fixation in patients unable to see the dot. A further variation in chart 3 has the same grid of red lines on black. These red squares may be useful in detecting colour desaturation in optic nerve disease.

How to do it

The test is performed as follows:

- Ensure adequate lighting conditions.
- Each eye is tested individually whilst wearing reading correction if required.
- The patient is asked to look at the centre dot on the chart and report any distortion, blurring or missing areas on the chart. Asking the patient to draw what is seen onto the chart provides a record for the case notes (Fig. 19.2).

Interpretation

- In general, patients with macular disease may report distortion (metamorphopsia) or blurring of the grid lines. Conversely, optic neuropathy may cause faintness of the chart or missing lines (scotoma).

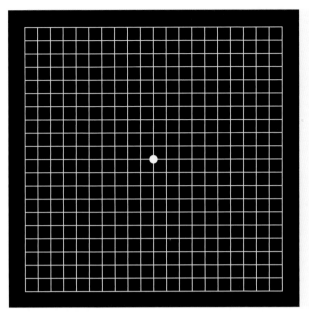

Fig. 19.1 Amsler grid chart (white on black). Most clinicians, however, use the Amsler grid recording chart (Fig. 19.2) to perform the test.

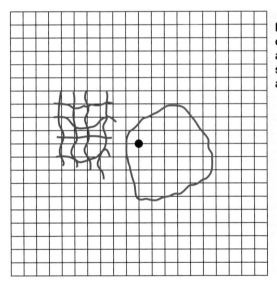

Fig. 19.2 Amsler grid recording chart (black on white) showing areas of metamorphopsia and scotoma perceived and drawn by a patient.

- Metamorphopsia is caused by disruption of the regular anatomical array of photoreceptors at the macula. This is usually due to macular oedema, whether secondary to retinal vascular disease (e.g. diabetic maculopathy, retinal venous occlusion) or choroidal vascular disease (e.g. exudative age-related maculopathy). Occasionally, metamorphopsia may be due to other macular pathology or disease further back in the visual pathway.

- Blurring of grid lines is caused by macular disease resulting in reduction of photoreceptor density. This causes reduced resolution of the image and therefore visual blurring.

20

B-scan ultrasound

JP Kersey

Introduction

This is a technique for examining the eye using a machine identical in principle to that used for obstetric ultrasound. Newer machines provide excellent resolution and use frequencies above 10 MHz. The higher the frequency of the ultrasound, the better the resolution, but the worse the penetration and so higher power is needed.

B-scan ultrasonography produces a dynamic two-dimensional cross-section of the eye and is typically used to examine the posterior segment when direct visualisation is not possible (e.g. in the presence of a dense vitreous haemorrhage or cataract). It is also often used to provide an objective measure of thickness of posterior segment lesions (e.g. choroidal naevi).

Principles

B-scan (or brightness mode) ultrasound represents the intensity of the ultrasound reflectivity signal as the brightness of the point on the scan, compared with the A-scan (amplitude mode—used in ocular biometry), which represents higher reflectance signals with a greater amplitude on the trace.

The machines either use a single oscillating piezoelectric crystal or an array of several crystals. These crystals vibrate with changes in electric current, so producing ultrasound waves, which then pass into the eye and are reflected from the interfaces of tissues with different conductivity. The time taken to return to the probe allows the distance from the probe to be calculated, and the amount of signal returning is shown by the intensity of the scan at that point.

How to do it

A B-scan can be performed with the eyelids closed (usually) or alternatively open (rarely, performed with generous topical anaesthesia). Gel is placed on the probe to improve ultrasound transmission and the probe placed on the eyelid. The probe is then moved over the lid to allow visualisation of different parts of the globe. The probe must be held perpendicular to the globe to maximise the amount of signal returning to the probe and so optimise image quality. White on the screen image represents high reflectivity, while black represents low reflectivity.

- The best-visualised target is the optic nerve, as the optic nerve head casts a dense acoustic shadow (a dark area behind the optic nerve head), as almost all the ultrasound signal is reflected.

- To find the optic nerve head and its characteristic acoustic shadow, hold the probe ≈15° temporally from the visual axis of the patient; it should now be pointing slightly towards the nasal retina. Areas of high reflectivity, such as retinal calcification, can also produce an acoustic shadow, which can appear similar to the optic nerve's appearance.

- The macular area can now be visualised by moving the probe over the surface of the lid to point along the visual axis.

- Systematic examination of the posterior pole can then be carried out by asking the patient to look in the four secondary positions of gaze (up, down, left and right) and angling the probe in the same direction. To examine the peripheral retina (e.g. at the three o'clock position) the patient is asked to look to the left and the probe tip is moved to the right (temporally), but with its axis pointing to the peripheral nasal retina.

- The examination is a dynamic process and the probe is gently rocked to perform sweeping views of the retina in that area.

- Most ultrasound probes have a mark on one side, which denotes the leading edge of the probe and the plane of the examination. The mark corresponds to the upper limit of the scan as shown on the screen. For example, if the probe is held with the mark in a vertical orientation, then the scan images seen on the screen will represent a vertical cross-section through the eye at that point.

- An initial examination is best done in the horizontal plane, allowing the horizontal extent of a lesion to be seen. The probe can then be rotated through 90° to provide a vertically orientated scan.

- Differentiating between retinal detachments and the posterior face of the vitreous can often be difficult and this requires a dynamic examination. A retinal detachment will always be attached at the optic disc while a vitreous detachment may well not be. On movement of the eye, vitreous detachments are usually far more mobile. To identify this, ask the patient to move the eye slightly to the left and then to the right to allow revisualisation of the lesion. The vitreous will be forced to move due to inertia and this can be seen on the ultrasound scan.

- Another common use for the B-scan is to measure the height of a choroidal or retinal lesion. This is particularly useful for suspected melanomas or in the monitoring of naevi. Machines have different methods of producing the measuring callipers and discussion with someone familiar with the machine will be needed.

- B-scan machines increasingly also have Doppler functions available, which can identify the degree of vascularity of a lesion. This is also useful in the examination of suspected melanomas as they have been reported to have a dual blood supply from both the retina and the choroid.

- The anterior chamber and lens are not clearly visible with the standard technique described above. To allow visualisation of these structures, an immersion technique or spacer, such as a bag of saline, must be used. This increases the distance from the cornea and allows adequate time for the ultrasound pulse to be emitted and received. Immersion A-scan ultrasound techniques are occasionally used to provide more accurate biometry information.

- The magnification of the scan image and the intensity (gain) of the scan can be altered. This often improves the visualisation of certain structures, while reducing the visualisation of others. Increasing the gain also increases the brightness of other structures within the eye, such as the vitreous, which may reduce the ability to discern the area of interest.

- To examine the optic nerve head, a low intensity image is usually needed, in contrast to examining the vitreous when a higher intensity may be required. The gain should be altered until an optimum visualisation of the area of interest is achieved.

- It is important to familiarise oneself with the equipment available before it is needed in the middle of the night on-call.

Other adaptations of the basic technique include ultrasound biomicroscopy (UBM). This allows very high-resolution images of the anterior segment to be obtained and has helped with the understanding of the pathophysiology of conditions such as the pigment dispersion syndrome (where iris position is thought to be relevant).

21

Worth's four dot test (Worth's lights)

MJ Hawker

Introduction

Worth's four dot test is a subjective orthoptic test used to investigate the state of retinal correspondence.

Principles

The test consists of four circular lights set in a diamond shape on a black/grey background (usually the light box of a Snellen chart)—one white, one red, and two green (Fig. 21.1). The patient wears red and green goggles, with the red goggle (which transmits red light and absorbs other wavelengths; = 'green filter') before the right eye. Viewing the lights through the filter glasses causes partial *dissociation*—the right eye sees the red light, the left eye sees the green lights, but both eyes see the white light, which therefore provides some stimulus for fusion. As a test of fusion in itself, Worth's lights provides little information because the targets are lights and are therefore gross, non-accommodative stimuli to fusion. A *prism fusion range test* or *synoptophore* provides much more information about the patient's fusional ability.

Worth's four lights can be used to test for:

- binocular single vision
- normal or abnormal retinal correspondence
- suppression
- diplopia.

Interpretation of the test requires knowledge of the results of cover testing performed on the patient (see Ch. 29).

How to do it

- Turn the room lights down (otherwise seeing other shapes in the room may stimulate fusion) and turn the test lights on. The test is first viewed from 6 m and then at 33 cm. When viewing the lights, the patient is asked how many are seen.
- If four lights are seen (the red, the two green, and the white appearing red/green), either there is normal *binocular single vision* or, if the patient has a manifest squint on cover testing (heterotropia), there is *abnormal retinal*

Ophthalmic equipment

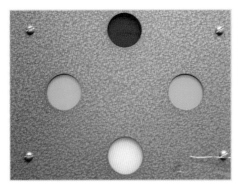

Fig 21.1 Worth's lights. These consist of a red light, two green lights and a white, presented on a grey or black background. In this case, they are mounted on the bottom of a standard light box.

correspondence (ARC). In ARC, the fovea of one eye develops a common visual direction with an extrafoveal element of the fellow eye.

- If two red lights only are seen (the red and the white) then *left suppression* is present.

- If three green lights only are seen (the two green and the white) then *right suppression* is present.

- If five lights are seen (two red and three green lights) then binocular single vision is absent and the patient has diplopia. If the two red lights are perceived to the left of the three green lights then the patient has a divergent squint (*exotropia*). Thus, the lights stimulate retinal elements temporal to the fovea and are projected into the nasal visual fields. If the two red lights are perceived to the right of the three green lights, then the patient has a convergent squint (*esotropia*).

- Viewing the lights at the two different distances helps to determine whether abnormalities affect near and distance vision equally.

Colour vision testing

MJ Hawker

Normal colour vision

The visible wavelengths of the electromagnetic spectrum are between 400 nm and 780 nm. Colour is perceived using signals from three populations of cone photoreceptors in the retina:

- 'blue' (*tritan*) cones maximally sensitive to short wavelengths (440 nm)
- 'green' (*deutan*) cones maximally sensitive to middle wavelengths (540 nm)
- 'red' (*protan*) cones maximally sensitive to long wavelengths (570 nm).

There is considerable overlap in the spectral sensitivities between these three types of photoreceptors. Normal colour vision requires the passage of light to the retina to be unchanged in spectral composition. Disease of the cornea, lens (e.g. yellow-tinged vision in nuclear sclerosis) and ocular media can all potentially change colour perception.

Colour vision defects

Problems with colour vision can be congenital or acquired.

Congenital defects occur if a cone pigment is absent or if there is a shift in its spectral sensitivity. *Deuteranopia, protanopia* and *tritanopia* indicate absence of green, red and blue cone function. *Deuteranomaly, protanomaly* and *tritanomaly* indicate altered spectral sensitivity in the corresponding cone and are much commoner. Congenital defects are much more common in males than females; the genes for red and green cones are carried by the X chromosome (therefore X-linked colour deficiencies). The blue pigment gene is found on chromosome 7. The prevalence of deuteranomaly in males (the most common defect) is around 5%; protanomaly, deuteranopia and protanopia prevalences are all around 1%, with congenital tritan defects being very uncommon. Monochromats, either with no cones (*achromatopsia*) or only one type of cone, are rare.

Of the acquired causes of colour vision defects, optic nerve disease tends to cause red/green defects, whereas acquired retinal disease tends to cause blue/yellow defects. There are exceptions to this rule, most notably glaucomatous optic neuropathy, which initially causes blue/yellow defects. A drug history is essential, as several drugs can cause colour vision shifts (e.g. *xanthopsia* in digoxin toxicity).

Ophthalmic equipment

Clinical testing of colour vision

Red desaturation

This is a quick and easy test for optic nerve dysfunction:

- Sit opposite the patient at a distance of about 1 m.
- Present a bright red object (e.g. red tip of hatpin) for the patient to observe with one eye at a time (ask the patient to cover the other eye).
- Relative dimness of the red colour in one eye compared with the other indicates red desaturation and may be caused by an optic nerve lesion.
- The same principle can be used to look for hemifield or quadrant field defects. Testing one eye at a time, ask the patient to look straight at your eye (patient's left eye looks straight at examiner's right eye and vice-versa).
- Hold up two bright red targets between yourself and the patient such that one target lies in the nasal hemifield and one in the temporal hemifield, but still within the central area of vision (and not the blind spot). Relative red desaturation of one target compared with the other may indicate early optic nerve disease (e.g. bitemporal red desaturation in the presence of a pituitary tumour compressing decussating nasal fibres).

Ishihara pseudoisochromatic plates (Fig. 22.1)

- Named after Shinobu Ishihara (1879–1963, Japan).
- Developed specifically as a screening test for congenital red/green defects (though it is commonly used to test for all red/green defects).
- A visual acuity of 6/18 or better is required to perform the test reliably.
- Consists of a series of plates, each with a matrix of coloured dots arranged so that a figure is only visible if colour vision is normal.
- The full test contains 38 plates, however, a shortened edition of 24 plates is commonly used.
- There are two groups of plates—the first group for numerates (25 plates towards the front of the book) and the second group for innumerates

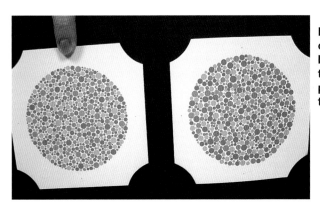

Fig. 22.1 Testing for congenital colour blindness using the Ishihara pseudoisochromatic test plates.

(13 plates towards the back of the book). The innumerate plates consist of winding paths to be traced by the patient. It is not necessary to use both types of plate on the same patient.

- There are different types of plates within the test (plate numbers for the 38 plate edition are given below).
  - Test plates (plates 1 and 38). The figures on these plates should be visible to all, regardless of colour vision, because the digits differ in contrast as well as colour.
  - Transformation plates (plates 2 to 9). Anomalous colour observers see different digits from those with normal colour vision.
  - Disappearing digit (vanishing) plates (plates 10 to 17). Only those with normal colour vision will see the digits.
  - Hidden digit plates (plates 18 to 21). Only those with anomalous colour vision will see the digits.
  - Qualitative plates (plates 22 to 25). These plates are intended to classify a congenital defect as protan or deutan, and as mild or severe.
- Of these different types, the transformation and vanishing plates (2 to 17) are the most reliable. Tests often use just these plates with scores marked out of 17 (test plate and these 16 plates).
- Table 22.1 shows what a normal person, a person with red/green deficiency and a person with total colour blindness (achromatopsia) should see when looking at each test plate in the 38 plate edition.

Performing the Ishihara test:
- Ensure adequate illumination in the room that does not cast a glare on the page (daylight if possible).
- The patient views the plates at reading distance (with reading correction if required) at an angle of 90°.
- If conducting the numerate test, start with the test plate (1st plate) and work forwards through the book. If conducting the innumerate test, start with the test plate at the back (38th plate) and work backwards through the book. If the patient cannot read the test plate, the whole test should be abandoned.
- Note the number of plates that are failed.
- A cut-off score of four failed plates is used (false positive rate of one-third in males, but higher than this in females).
- If the test is failed, formal testing using the D15 or Farnsworth–Munsell 100-hue test should follow.

Farnsworth–Munsell 100-hue test

- Detects and distinguishes all types of colour vision insufficiency from the mildest red/green defect to total achromatopsia.
- Although named the 100-hue test, it actually consists of 84 movable coloured tiles arranged in four boxes of 21 tiles each.
- The patient is given one tray at a time and is asked to arrange the coloured tiles in serial order of hue (chromatic order) between two reference tiles. This task is repeated for each tray.

Ophthalmic equipment

Table 22.1 What the normal person, the person with red/green deficiency, and the person with total colour blindness will see when looking at each test plate of the Ishihara test (38 plate edition)

Number of plate	Normal person	Person with red/green deficiency				Person with total colour blindness
1	12	12				12
2	8	3				Nil
3	6	5				Nil
4	29	70				Nil
5	57	35				Nil
6	5	2				Nil
7	3	5				Nil
8	15	17				Nil
9	74	21				Nil
10	2	Nil				Nil
11	6	Nil				Nil
12	97	Nil				Nil
13	45	Nil				Nil
14	5	Nil				Nil
15	7	Nil				Nil
16	16	Nil				Nil
17	73	Nil				Nil
18	X	5				Nil
19	X	2				Nil
20	X	45				Nil
21	X	73				Nil
		Protan		**Deutan**		
		Strong	**Mild**	**Strong**	**Mild**	
22	26	6	(2)6	2	2(6)	
23	42	2	(4)2	4	4(2)	
24	35	5	(3)5	3	3(5)	
25	96	6	(9)6	9	9(6)	

- The type and severity of abnormality in colour vision is determined by the position of any errors and their frequency. Results are plotted on a chart to visually display the errors.
- The test is time-consuming to perform and is not therefore suitable as a screening test.

Farnsworth–Munsell D15 test

- Consists of 15 loose tiles and one fixed (reference) tile displaying different hues. The differences in hue between each tile are approximately the same. When arranged in order, the tiles form a hue circle.
- Errors in the order of arrangement of the hues by the patient indicate colour deficiencies that can be interpreted on a chart.
- It is not designed as a screening test.
- The test will not separate anomalous trichromats from dichromats.

Automated visual field testing

JP Kersey

Introduction

The automated visual field analyser is extensively used in the glaucoma clinic. Clinical visual field testing by confrontation (see Ch. 26) is unreliable because it is subjective, crude, poorly reproducible and employs non-standardised conditions (e.g. variable levels of room lighting and different stimuli). It is unreliable at determining subtle field defects in one examination, let alone determining changes in field defects over time. Automation of visual field testing has improved accuracy, speed, reliability and reproducibility of testing beyond measure. Ophthalmologists and optometrists use field analysers daily and a good working knowledge of the tests is essential.

Principles

Retinal sensitivity to visual stimuli (measured in decibels) varies throughout the visual field, being highest at the fovea and lower in the periphery (and absent at the blind spot). Thus, the cross-sectional contour of retinal sensitivity is known as the 'hill of vision'. There are many different types of equipment for visual field testing (*perimetry*), but they fall into two main groups:

- *static* perimetry—e.g. Humphrey machine
- *dynamic* perimetry—e.g. Goldmann machine.

Static perimetry uses stationary targets (lights) of varying intensity to measure retinal sensitivity throughout the visual field being tested (commonly the central 24° or 30°). There are two main static perimetry test strategies:

- *Suprathreshold tests* employ stimuli of an intensity (measured in apostilbs) greater than the visual threshold that a normal person is able to detect. Such test strategies are used as screening tests for defects.
- *Threshold tests* take longer to perform as they map the threshold retinal sensitivity (stimulus intensity below which the light is not detected) at many points across the visual field. Threshold tests detect more subtle differences in field size and shape and are often used to chart progression of glaucomatous field loss (as defects often deepen before they enlarge).

The *Estermann visual field test* is performed by the Humphrey machine and uses static stimuli to examine the binocular visual field. It is used to check that patients fulfil the Driver and Vehicle Licensing Agency requirements to drive (see Ch. 61).

Dynamic perimetry (e.g. Goldmann perimetry) tests retinal sensitivity to a moving target (usually a light). The specific target size and intensity may be varied to map out the limits of the visual field to that particular target. Dynamic perimetry detects less subtle defects than static perimetry and is often used to detect neurological field changes. It is more difficult for the ophthalmologist to perform than static perimetry (in that it is not truly automated and requires an operator), but provides information about the periphery of the visual fields unobtainable with static perimetry. Furthermore, the fact that Goldmann perimetry is not automated means that visual field examination can be customised to provide detailed information about the midline, blind spot, etc. An understanding of how to perform static and dynamic perimetry is a requirement of the current Royal College Part II Examination.

Humphrey machine

The machine initially identifies the blind spot and then starts to present the main field lights. If the light is seen then it will present a much dimmer light until the target is not seen. If the target is not seen, a brighter light will be presented. This will be repeated until the threshold level has been established. The machine also runs spot checks within the blind spot to ensure that fixation has not moved (fixation rate). Lights above an established threshold are used to establish concentration (false negative rate); over-enthusiasm (false positive rate) is monitored by the machine making the audible click that normally accompanies a stimulus, but without a light stimulus per se.

The Humphrey has many different protocols, but the following are most commonly used:

- Central 76: a suprathreshold test of the central 30 degrees of visual field. Commonly used as a screening test and especially useful for neurological defects.

- 24-2: a threshold test of the central 24 degrees of visual field (commonly used in monitoring glaucoma patients).

- 10-2: a threshold test of the central 10 degrees of visual field. This is a specific test for central scotomata and monitoring fixation-threatening disease, e.g. in advanced glaucoma.

SITA fast is a software program, which uses a Swedish testing algorithm to minimise the number of test spots needed to produce an accurate field test plot. It has effectively halved the field test times.

Statpac is a statistical package, which analyses the field test results and forms the usual printout for most hospitals' Humphrey machines. The upper printout represents the actual numerical thresholds and also has a graphical representation in a grey scale. These are of limited value as they are not a comparison with normal values. The two lower plots are: total deviation, a comparison of the basic data with an age-matched normal field; and pattern deviation which also takes into account overall changes in threshold, such as cataracts.

Ophthalmic equipment

Global indices

- MD (mean deviation) is the mean difference between the measured field and the age-corrected normal reference field.
- PSD (pattern standard deviation) is a measurement of the difference in shape between the measured field and the age-matched normal field, a high number indicating an irregular hill of vision.
- SF (short-term fluctuation) is measured by rechecking ten pre-selected points to check the patient's consistency.
- CPSD (corrected pattern standard deviation) is a measure of how much the total shape of the hill of vision differs from the normal age-matched hill shape, corrected for the short-term fluctuations (above).

Humphrey—how to do it

- Enter the patient's details into the computer (including age, in order to facilitate analysis by comparison with age-specific normal visual fields).
- Ask the patient to place chin on the rest and adjust the height of the patient and chin rest to optimise comfort (the test can last up to 10 minutes depending on the protocol used).
- If the patient requires glasses to read they should be worn for the test (not bifocals or varifocals). Alternatively, suitable *plus* lenses can be placed in the holder on the machine. The eyes are tested individually (contralateral eye covered with a patch).
- The patient is told to maintain fixation on a small white central light. This is encouraged throughout the test—fixation losses considerably reduce the reliability of the test.
- Start the test.
- The patient presses a button each time they see a light shine (somewhere in the visual field).

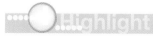

Static perimetry: tips and pitfalls

- If the lids are droopy or the lens is not close to the eye, artefacts will be produced.
- When comparing visual fields over time it helps to maintain the same test protocol each time. This makes it much easier to interpret changes.
- Only the DVLA can say categorically whether a driving field test is adequate. They do, however, publish their criteria for license based on Estermann visual field testing.

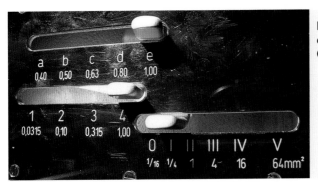

Fig. 23.1 Control levers on the console of the Goldmann perimeter.

Goldmann

This machine requires some practice to be able to get reliable visual fields from the patient. A target stimulus (light) of specific size and brightness is selected using the levers shown (Fig. 23.1). I (size) 4e (brightness) is the commonest starting target. If this is not detected at all, a brighter and/or larger target is used.

There are six different possible size settings, each being four times larger than the next smallest target: e.g. '0' is 0.0625 mm², 'I' is 0.25 mm², and so on to 'V', being 64 mm². The brightness of the target is measured in decibels or apostilbs, which can be adjusted in steps according to the scale on each individual Goldmann machine (4 to 1, and e, d, c, b, a).

Goldmann—how to do it

- Ask the patient to place chin on the rest and ensure a reading correction is used if appropriate (Fig. 23.2). Insert a Goldmann visual field recording chart into the holder and tighten the fixing screws.

- Instruct the patient to maintain gaze on the central target (usually a light). A telescope at the back of the machine enables the examiner to check fixation.

- The target light is moved manually in from the periphery (using levers) until it is seen by the patient. When first detected, the patient taps the table or presses a buzzer.

- Once the target has been seen, the position of the threshold is marked on the recording chart (Fig. 23.3). The light is moved to another meridian and the test repeated, until all meridia have been tested. The points at which the light was first seen are joined together to produce a threshold line (*isopter*).

- Due to the slightly antiquated design of the Goldmann machine, it is important to be careful to follow the instructions on the recording chart when moving across the horizontal midline (Fig. 23.4).

Ophthalmic equipment

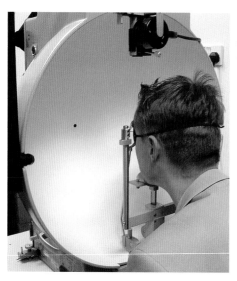

Fig. 23.2 Patient in position at Goldmann machine. Place a patch over one of the patient's eyes and ask the patient to place chin into the test bowl.

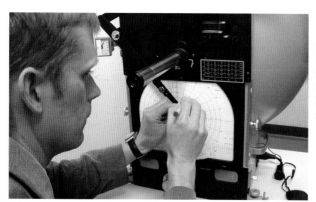

Fig. 23.3 Goldmann machine. When a stimulus is seen for the first time, mark its position on the recording chart (part of the isopter for this particular stimulus type).

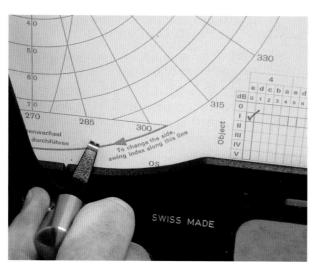

Fig. 23.4 Changing sides on the Goldmann machine. Follow the instructions on the recording chart to avoid damaging the machine.

- The test is then repeated with a dimmer or smaller target to produce a second threshold line within the first (this represents a higher contour on the hill of vision).

- The blind spot also needs to be separately plotted as it may well fall between the two thresholds measured.

Highlight

Goldmann: tips and pitfalls

- Central scotomata are best mapped with a red target and need to be examined for specifically, as they will often be within the previous threshold lines.

- Fixation should be checked regularly to ensure a reliable test.

Heidelberg retinal tomography (HRT)

BJ McDermott

Introduction

Recent advances in the understanding of the aetiology and progression of glaucoma have led to the realisation that change in the appearance of the optic disc is of vital importance. The ability to objectively recognise such changes is essential to aid both diagnosis and management. Examination of the optic disc with a 78 or 90 D lens has previously been supported with optic disc photography, but, in recent years, examination of the disc with laser technology has become available, with built-in software enabling progression analysis over serial images. Systems include: laser optical cross-sectioning, scanning laser polarimetry, low coherence interferometry and scanning laser tomography. HRT II is a scanning laser tomograph that is a version of a previous research tool (HRT I), which has been modified for clinical use.

Principles

The HRT II consists of the following parts:

- computer
- laser scanning camera
- patient headrest
- operating software.

The HRT II is a confocal laser scanning system, which allows the acquisition and analysis of three-dimensional images of the optic disc. It produces measurements (in microns) of the disc area, rim and cup areas, rim and cup volumes and rim/disc area ratio. Measurements of the retinal nerve fibre layer immediately surrounding the disc are also given. These measurements are produced for the whole disc, and also for six predefined sectors (temporal, temporal-superior, temporal-inferior, and similarly for the nasal disc). Its most important application is to detect glaucomatous damage to the optic nerve head (loss of rim) and in the follow-up of glaucomatous progression. The HRT II can detect subtle changes in the optic nerve head in advance of visual field deterioration. It does this by comparing the actual rim area with that predicted by the Moorfields Regression Analysis. At the time of writing, this is based on a database of 112 eyes, and predicts rim area corrected for age and disc area. As disc area increases, sensitivity is known to rise although at the expense of specificity. The software also quantifies change in optic nerve head morphology over time.

The examination

The patient having an HRT II examination does not require special preparation, and it is generally possible to perform the test without pupil dilation; occasionally, dilation may be required in the presence of media opacities such as cataracts. As a general rule, the image is acquired without the patient wearing glasses, as refractive variations of up to 12 D can be adjusted for using the lens on the camera. If a patient has astigmatism greater than 1 D, they can wear glasses or contact lenses; alternatively, an additional set of corrective cylindrical lenses can be purchased for use with the machine. HRT II examination is best carried out prior to tonometry or the installation of any ointment or fluorescein.

How to do it

- Ask the patient to sit comfortably with the head on the rest and the chin and forehead firmly forward in the frame.
- Ask the patient to blink two or three times and then to fixate on the green flashing light found within the camera structure.
- Dial the lens adjustment to create as clear an image as possible of the optic nerve head on the display screen.
- Ask the patient to blink again a few times and then to stare at the fixation light without blinking or moving.
- Push the laser button to commence the scanning. The scanning process only takes a few seconds to perform.
- The process can then be repeated for the fellow eye.
- Look at the images on screen and assess their quality by looking at the picture and by referring to the standard deviation of the image value. Standard deviations less than 20 generally indicate high quality images.
- If necessary, another set of images can be undertaken and the best ones used. For all baseline examinations, it is recommended to acquire two sets of images.

The rest can be done without the patient present. It is possible to view a movie of the image acquisition and to see the topography on screen as a three-dimensional image. These are both very helpful before the examiner draws the contour line around the optic disc margin, which is done using the mouse. A good knowledge of the basics of optic disc anatomy is obviously a prerequisite for recognising the disc margin and hence being able to draw a reliable contour line (unfortunately, the computer is unable to do this for you). Once the disc margin contour line has been drawn, the software calculates the disc measurements described above. The software transfers the same contour line on to subsequent images. If the contour is redrawn on a subsequent examination then it will affect the results both retrospectively and prospectively. Once done, the HRT II will automatically make an assessment of the optic nerve head, divide it into the six segments and classify each segment according to the Moorfields regression analysis as: 'Within normal limits', 'Borderline' or 'Outside normal limits' (Figs 24.1 and 24.2).

Ophthalmic equipment

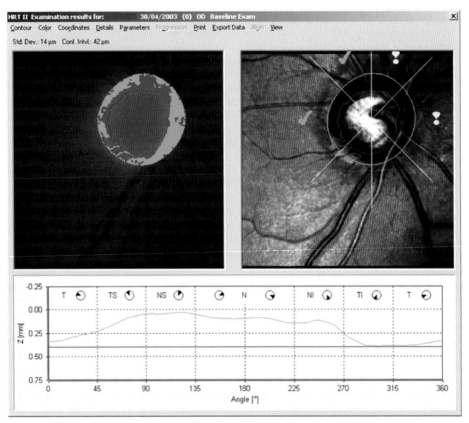

Fig. 24.1 HRT II results: image of the optic nerve head taken using the Heidelberg retina tomograph (II). The software displays the height profile of the retinal nerve fibre layer along the optic disc contour.

Which patients?

The HRT II is best used for glaucoma suspects that are deemed to be 'high risk' and for those patients with early glaucoma. In patients with advanced glaucoma, where the neuroretinal rim is severely compromised, HRT probably has less application. The frequency of scanning depends on the perceived rate of progression. For a small number of patients who cannot perform visual field tests well, the HRT II may be the best way of monitoring their condition, but it has to be borne in mind that some patients may not be able to comply with the demands of the test. Note also that the Moorfields regression analysis used a sample of patients with a mean age of 57 years. How the analysis handles elderly patients (the majority with glaucoma) has not been confirmed.

The HRT II will not give useful results if the ocular media are not clear, if there is a high degree of astigmatism that cannot be overcome with lenses, or if the patient is unable to fixate well, such as in advanced macular disease where patients may find it difficult to locate the green pinpoint light. If you are in doubt as to whether or not a patient is suitable, it is often best to request the test and the HRT II operator will soon inform you if it is not appropriate!

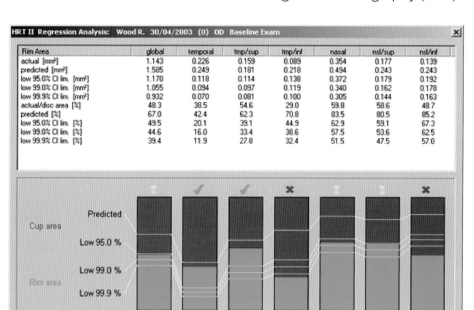

Rim Area	global	temporal	tmp/sup	tmp/inf	nasal	nsl/sup	nsl/inf
actual [mm²]	1.143	0.226	0.159	0.089	0.354	0.177	0.139
predicted [mm²]	1.585	0.249	0.181	0.218	0.494	0.243	0.243
low 95.0% CI lim. [mm²]	1.170	0.118	0.114	0.138	0.372	0.179	0.192
low 99.0% CI lim. [mm²]	1.055	0.094	0.097	0.119	0.340	0.162	0.178
low 99.9% CI lim. [mm²]	0.932	0.070	0.081	0.100	0.305	0.144	0.163
actual/disc area [%]	48.3	38.5	54.6	29.0	59.8	58.6	48.7
predicted [%]	67.0	42.4	62.3	70.8	83.5	80.5	85.2
low 95.0% CI lim. [%]	49.5	20.1	39.1	44.9	62.9	59.1	67.3
low 99.0% CI lim. [%]	44.6	16.0	33.4	38.6	57.5	53.6	62.5
low 99.9% CI lim. [%]	39.4	11.9	27.8	32.4	51.5	47.5	57.0

Fig. 24.2 HRT II results: the Moorfields regression analysis compares the actual rim area with that predicted for an optic disc of this particular size and age. A green tick marks rim area 'Within normal limits', with a red cross indicating 'Outside normal limits' and a yellow '!' symbol indicating 'Borderline'.

What the HRT II can tell you

The HRT II can provide a number of on-screen result displays or hard copies to be filed within the patient's notes. In addition to the parameters described above, it is also possible to make interactive measurements across the image, including height and position measurements. Printable reports include the baseline images, standard report and Moorfields regression analysis. For subsequent examination, progression analysis, the stereometric progression chart and a trend report is available. Clearly, the more examinations accrued, the more helpful it can become and any past images that were not so perfect can be dropped out, so allowing for more accurate results.

Section 3
Examination of patients

Visual acuity

JP Kersey

Distance acuity charts

Distance visual acuity (VA) is a fundamental part of every ophthalmic examination. It should be performed at every visit, with glasses if appropriate, and with a pinhole (if the measured VA is suboptimal).

There are two main standards at present (Snellen and LogMAR), both based on the reading of letter charts.

Snellen chart (Fig. 25.1)

The patient most commonly stands 6 m from the chart, though smaller charts for closer test distances are available (see the inside back cover for an end-of-bed Snellen chart). Patients read the chart usually with their refraction corrected (e.g. with spectacles on) and then through a pinhole. It is easy and quick to perform, however, it is poor at noting small changes, especially with lower acuities.

The chart starts with a single big letter at the top, with the letters decreasing in size as one progresses down the chart; as the letters are smaller further down the chart, more letters are present on each line. For patients who are unable to read, the 'illiterate E' chart may be used (usually one of the sides of a Snellen light box); for each of the 'E's, which decrease in size as one reads down the chart, the patient must decide in which direction the limbs of the 'E' are pointing.

The Snellen notation is in the form of a fraction of ideal vision. The upper figure is the distance at which the chart is being viewed by the patient and the lower figure is the smallest line on the chart that they can read. This lower figure represents the furthest distance from the chart that a patient with normal acuity could stand to read that particular line correctly. This is also the distance from the eye at which each bar or space of the target (e.g. the height of each limb of a letter 'E') would subtend an angle of 1 minute of arc ($\frac{1}{60}$ of a degree) on the retina. For example:

- 6/6 = normal vision (20/20 in America, as they use feet rather than metres).
- 3/60 = very poor vision (as it means a patient standing 3 m from the chart can only read letters which a person with normal vision could read if they were 60 m away).

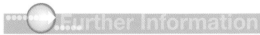

Further Information

The crowding effect

The crowding effect increases as one moves down the chart. This is due to the increased number of letters on the lower lines and differentially affects amblyopic eyes more than normals (such that visual acuity is underestimated more in amblyopia).

Examination of patients

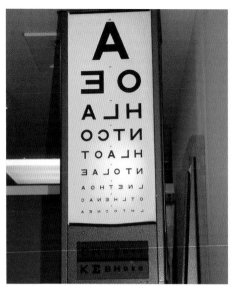

Fig. 25.1 A light box with a Snellen chart for testing distance vision (6 m). This chart is inverted, requiring the use of a mirror (at 3 m) to see correctly.

LogMAR charts, e.g. ETDRS chart (Bailey–Lovie chart) (Fig. 25.2)

Made popular by the 'Early treatment diabetic retinopathy study' as the gold standard for research, this is based on a logarithmic approach. Each line on the chart is smaller than the previous by a fixed proportion. This method attempts to produce a continuous acuity score. Depending on the particular sized chart involved (3 m chart, 4 m chart, etc.), the patient stands at that distance from the chart, wearing the appropriate spectacle correction.

There are ten lines between 6/60 (score 1.0) and 6/6 (score 0.0) equivalents. Each line contains five letters and each letter carries a value of 0.02. A decimal score is produced, from 0.0 to 1.0 (for better and worse vision, negative scores and scores greater than 1.0 are produced) as follows. For each full line the patient reads, 0.1 (= 5 × 0.02) is subtracted from 1.0. When they are not able to read a complete line, 0.02 for each letter read correctly is then subtracted and the test ends.

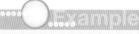

LogMAR

If the patient could read the first 8 lines, and 3 letters correctly from the next line, they would score:

$$1.0 - (8 \times 0.1) - (3 \times 0.02) = 1.0 - 0.8 - 0.06 = 1.0 - 0.86 = 0.14$$

The test does take slightly longer to perform than the Snellen chart, however, it is increasing in popularity and is more useful in research.

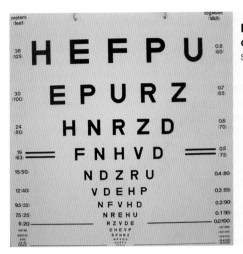

Fig. 25.2 An example of a logMAR chart. Note that each line contains the same number of letters.

The pinhole effect

The pinhole acts to reduce the light entering the eye to a small beam. This removes the need to focus the light beam, so acting to compensate for refractive errors (up to several dioptres only) and causes of glare such as corneal scarring or cataract. It is a very useful test to differentiate between organic pathology, which is not improved with a pinhole, and refractive error, which may be.

Near acuity charts

These test a subject's near vision and use one of several reading type charts (see inside back cover for N near vision chart). These charts have a series of paragraphs with increasingly smaller text. The patient reads the smallest text they can comfortably, with each eye individually, while wearing the appropriate refractive correction. Near vision is generally held to be more sensitive than distance acuity for changes in acuity due to macular disease.

The Jaeger chart scores the near vision by a J score (arbitrary numbers); J6 is small type while J20 is larger type (poor vision).

Other charts use the British N score, where each point is equivalent to 1/72 of an inch of total height of the letters: N4.5 is usually the smallest available.

Binocular visual acuity

This is a test of binocular single vision and involves asking the patient to read reducing letter sizes, such as those of either the Snellen or LogMAR charts, at both 6 m (distance) and $\frac{1}{3}$ m (near). A cover/uncover test (see Ch. 29) is performed during the test in order to identify whether binocular single vision is being maintained. If a manifest squint develops, then the binocular visual acuity is recorded as the previously completed line.

Examination of patients

Testing visual acuity in children

There are many different methods available, each with difficulties. Orthoptists are the most expert at testing visual acuity in children, and are often an invaluable resource (particularly in dealing with children younger than three years of age). The reading acuity of children is very attention-dependent and a single acuity measure needs to be interpreted with caution.

The descriptions in Table 25.1 are designed to give you an idea of what is available and what age group the individual tests suit best. There are, of course, exceptions and not all children develop their visual or language functions at the same time. The chosen test does need to be appropriate for the verbal reasoning and language ability of the child being tested.

Table 25.1 Recommended visual acuity tests for specific age groups of children

Age range	Recommended tests
0–3 months	Facial recognition, CSM*, optokinetic nystagmus (see Ch. 30), visual-evoked potentials (see Ch. 40)
3–6 months	Visually directed reaching, Catford drum, preferential looking tests
6–12 months	Worth's static and rolling balls, small sweet tests (e.g. 'hundreds & thousands')
1–2 years	Kay's pictures, STYCAR ('Screening Test for Young Children And Retards'), Cardiff cards
3–5 years	Sheridan–Gardiner, Landolt's broken rings, Sonksten–Silver
6 years +	Snellen, ETDRS logMAR chart, N tests, J tests

*CSM (central, steady and maintained) involves covering one eye while the child is fixating on an object (toy). The non-covered eye should remain with central fixation, steady in its position and maintained through a blink. It is a good gross test for fixation ability.

Visual field testing by confrontation

SN Madge

Introduction

The following is a suggested technique for examining the visual fields of a patient in clinical practice; in addition, it may be useful as a checklist for candidates preparing for Examinations such as Part II of the MRCOphth Examination.

It should be stated at this point that, although relatively gross visual field defects can usually be picked up with good clinical skills, a more formal examination of a patient (e.g. Goldmann or Humphrey fields, see Ch. 23) is recommended in the clinic setting to avoid missing more subtle defects, as well as providing a definitive and objective record of the findings. By definition, confrontational visual fields require the examiner to have normal fields, or at least be aware of what is normal, as the examiner is being directly compared to the patient.

How to do it

- Particularly in Examinations, introduce yourself clearly to the patient and explain in simple terms what you are doing and exactly what you want the patient to do.

- Sit down approximately 1 m from and directly opposite the patient (knees just touching is a useful judge). Try and ensure that you are on a similar level to the patient.

- Consider the visual acuity of the eyes (or ask the Examiner)—if there is very poor sight, consider using a different stimulus for testing than the hatpins suggested below.

- First test for spatial neglect. Having asked the patient to keep both eyes open and fixate on your nose, hold out your arms to each side. Ask the patient to 'point to the hand that you see wiggling'. First wiggle the fingers of one hand, then the other, and then finally both together. In the presence of visual neglect, the responses to individual movements will be intact (i.e. no hemianopia), but only movements ipsilateral to the responsible parietal lesion will be detected when bilateral simultaneous movements are presented.

- Then test the visual fields of each eye in turn, initially using a white pin (typically 5 mm diameter).

- Cover your right eye with the palm of your hand and ask the patient to cover his or her left eye in a similar fashion. Ask the patient to stare into your eye, and instruct the patient to say 'yes' as soon as the pin becomes visible

Examination of patients

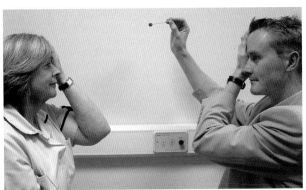

Fig. 26.1 Examining the visual field of a patient. Note that the examiner and patient are on the same level, approximately 1 m apart and that the stimulus (red pin in this example) is carefully held halfway between patient and examiner.

(Fig. 26.1); also instruct the patient to say 'gone' if the pin subsequently disappears as the test continues (e.g. in the presence of a dense central scotoma).

- Map out the four quadrants for each eye, remembering that the quadrants run from 12 o'clock to 3 o'clock, 3 o'clock to 6 o'clock and so forth; there is no discriminative value in testing along the 12, 3, 6 or 9 o'clock meridia themselves.

- Start from the periphery where the pin is outside the normal visual field and gradually move centrally. Even if the patient has said 'yes', keep moving the pin towards the centre in order to detect a central scotoma. If defects are found, attempt to map out these defects, especially along horizontal or vertical borders.

- Map out the peripheral field of the other eye and compare defects between the two eyes. In particular look for homonymous or bitemporal patterns.

- If the peripheral visual field is normal, it is still possible that there is a central visual field defect. This may often be detected by use of the red pin (again typically 5 mm diameter). Ask the patient to cover the respective eye in the usual fashion and say to the patient something like: 'this is a red pin, although you might not always see it as red as I move it around. Please say "red" as soon as you see the pin as red and not when you first see the pin. Remember to keep staring into my eye throughout the test.' Again, start from the periphery in all four quadrants, bringing the pin towards the centre as previously. Then repeat for the other eye. In the presence of an early bitemporal hemianopia, there will be reduced perception of the pin as red in the temporal field of each eye as compared with the nasal field.

- Test the size of the patient's blind spot by comparing it with your own in the four principal meridia (Fig. 26.2). Do this with the red pin, asking the patient to say 'gone' when the pin disappears and 'back' when it comes back or reappears. Compare the blind spot in the two eyes.

- Finally, test for temporal red desaturation if no defects have been found thus far. Occlude one eye as previously described and hold up two red pins: one immediately in the visual axis for the patient and another a few centimetres temporal to this. Ensure that the pin does not fall within the patient's blind spot. Ask the patient whether the two pins appear to be the same colour or

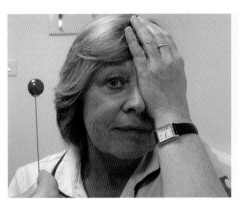

Fig. 26.2 Testing the blind spot. With the patient fixating your eye (and vice versa), move the red pin slowly in the temporal field of vision until the patient finds it disappears. Compare your blind spot with the patient's in terms of size and shape. Remember to keep the pin equidistant between you both.

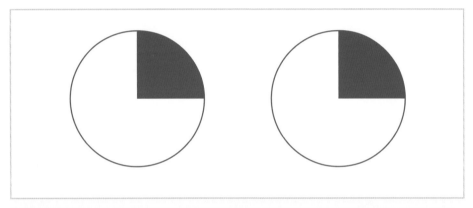

Fig 26.3 Documentation of a right superior homonymous quadrantanopia. With the patient's right eye being documented on the right side of the notes.

whether there is a difference (usually less red, or even black) between the two. A difference may represent chiasmal compression and a developing bitemporal hemianopia, particularly if substantiated in the other eye.

- In an Examination, offer thanks to the patient and then tell the Examiner that you would like to confirm your findings using a Goldmann perimeter (if appropriate). Consider whether ophthalmoscopic examination of the optic nerve may be helpful (e.g. in papilloedema and associated enlarged blind spot).

- In the clinic setting, document your findings in the notes. These are usually drawn from the patient's perspective but are also labelled clearly (right eye on right side of page, left eye on left; Fig. 26.3).

Examination of ptosis

MJ Hawker

Introduction

Ptosis (drooping of the eyelid) is observed commonly in clinical practice. Although most are due to age-related or involutional changes of the levator complex, there is a wide range of potential causes that might be missed if not specifically looked for.

A thorough assessment of ptosis includes taking a history, examination and, in certain cases, further investigations.

History

Ask about the following:

- duration/age of onset (congenital or acquired)
- family history (e.g. blepharophimosis syndrome)
- past history: type of delivery (forceps trauma), other trauma. Related medical conditions, e.g. myasthenia gravis, myotonia, myopathy, muscular dystrophy
- associated symptoms:
    - diplopia (III palsy/aberrant regeneration, trauma)
    - jaw-winking (Marcus Gunn syndrome)
    - fatigue during day (myasthenia gravis, levator weakness compensated for by Muller's muscle, which fatigues)
    - dysphagia (oculopharyngeal muscular dystrophy)
    - ophthalmoplegia (Kearns–Sayre syndrome)
- drug history (topical steroids, neostigmine)
- contact lens wear (can induce ptosis).

Examination

Observe the patient for:

- ptosis (unilateral or bilateral)
- strabismus (III palsy, myasthenia)
- frontalis overaction (raised eyebrows to compensate)

- local trauma (eyelid scars)
- mechanical causes (tumour on eyelid)
- pseudoptosis (e.g. ipsilateral microphthalmos or hypertropia, contralateral lid retraction or proptosis)
- pupils (III palsy, Horner's syndrome).

Using a clear plastic ruler, perform the following measurements to characterise the ptosis (see Fig. 27.1):

- Middle palpebral distance (or aperture, mm): vertical distance between upper and lower lid margins in the middle. Measure with the patient looking straight ahead (present a pen torch to fixate on).
- Marginal reflex distance (mm):
  - Distance between the corneal light reflex and lid margin.
  - Measure to upper (and lower lid) margins.
  - The middle palpebral distance may be equal bilaterally if there is lower lid ectropion in the eye with ptosis.
- Skin crease = distance (mm) between upper lid margin and upper lid horizontal skin crease:

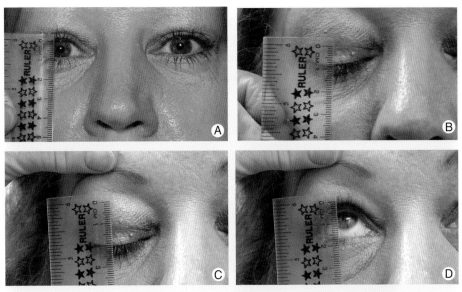

Fig. 27.1 Measurements to characterise ptosis. A. Measurement of the margin reflex distance (MRD) and middle palpebral aperture (PA) of the right eye. The distance from the reflex to the upper lid is the MRD (4 mm here) and the distance between the middle of the lids is the PA (8 mm here). **B.** Measurement of the skin crease. This is the distance from the upper lid crease to the bottom of the upper lid (8 mm here). **C & D.** Measurement of levator function. It is easy to overestimate levator function if the brow is not immobilised. Then measure the excursion of the upper lid from downgaze to upgaze (≈16 mm in this case).

Examination of patients

- The skin crease is formed by the insertion of the levator aponeurosis.
- Normal skin crease distance is 6–8 mm in males and 8–10 mm in females.
- A high crease may be seen in aponeurotic defects with normal levator function.
- Levator function = distance the upper lid margin travels on full excursion from downgaze to upgaze (mm).
  - Place a firm thumb above the eyebrow to immobilise frontalis muscle.
  - Ask the patient to look fully down then fully up, measuring the distance the upper lid margin moves.
  - Normal > 15 mm, good > 12 mm, fair > 5 mm, poor < 5 mm.

Further examination

- Assess lid closure and Bell's phenomenon (ask the patient to look down, hold the upper lid up, and ask the patient to close the eyes—the eyeball should roll up to protect the cornea under the upper lid; Fig. 27.2). If surgery for ptosis is contemplated, a poor Bell's reflex contributes to the risk of causing corneal exposure.
- Test corneal sensation with a drawn-out wisp of cotton wool. Ask the patient to look away from the direction you are approaching from and stroke the wisp directly across the cornea, without touching the conjunctiva first. Compare sensation between eyes. Reduced corneal sensation is a risk factor for exposure keratopathy after ptosis surgery.
- Assess fatigue—ask the patient to look up for 60 seconds. If the eyelids fatigue and droop, this suggests myasthenia.
- Cogan's twitch—seen in myasthenia. As the patient saccades between a downward target and the primary position, the upper lid overshoots when gaze returns to the primary position.
- Aberrant eyelid movements:
  - Marcus Gunn jaw-winking (ask the patient to move the jaw from side to side, or provide a sweet to chew—aberrant lid movements are seen with the jaw movement)

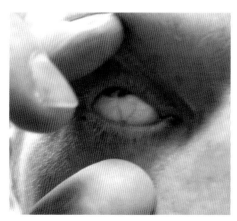

Fig. 27.2 An example of Bell's phenomenon.

- aberrant III regeneration—eyelid movements are seen with eye movements (e.g. medial rectus action).
- Test ocular movements, including saccades:
  - aberrant III regeneration, myasthenic ophthalmoplegia, chronic progressive external ophthalmoplegia
  - congenital ptosis can have superior rectus weakness.
- Test the pupillary reactions:
  - Horner's syndrome
  - III palsy.
- Check the fundus: Kearns–Sayre pigmentary retinopathy.

Further investigations

- Ice test (for myasthenia). Measure the middle palpebral distance before and after placement of ice (over a cloth) on the eyelids. An increase of 2 mm or more is a positive test. The cold temperature reduces metabolism of acetylcholine (ACh), thereby overcoming the low ACh receptor density.
- Tensilon test (best done by a neurologist).
- Anti-ACh receptor antibodies.
- Electromyography.

Examination of the pupils

SN Madge

Introduction

Pupillary abnormalities are not only common in clinical practice, but often also feature in clinical examinations. The following is a widely accepted routine for examination of the pupillary reflexes.

Remember that two distinct pupillary abnormalities may coexist within the same patient. For example, physiological *anisocoria* (a difference in pupil size between the two eyes) is very common and, if found in association with a relative afferent pupillary defect, it may lead to confusion in the inexperienced clinician.

How to do it

- General inspection:
    - Note first the lighting conditions of the room. In relative darkness, the abnormal eye is likely to have the smaller pupil (as a normal pupil would have undergone dilatation). Conversely, in bright conditions, the abnormal eye is likely to have the larger pupil (as a normal pupil would have constricted).
    - Inspect carefully for *heterochromia* (congenital Horner's syndrome), general position of the eye (*pseudoenophthalmos*, Horner's; *strabismus*, e.g. 'down-and-out' 3rd nerve palsy) and ptosis (3rd nerve palsy or Horner's syndrome).
- *Preparation.* In good light, ask the patient to fix on a distant target. Compare the pupil sizes (is anisocoria obvious?) and shape (are the pupils regular?). Is there obvious evidence of previous surgery (may lead to fixed *mydriasis*)? Sit to one side of the patient and hold the torch close to each eye in turn, but not obscuring the patient's gaze (may otherwise stimulate near response, see below). Then dim the lights.
- *Test the direct pupillary response in each eye in turn.* Ensure that the patient maintains distant fixation throughout. Observe the pupillary constriction seen in response to light shone in the same eye. If there is a suspicion of Horner's syndrome (small pupil, difference more marked in the dark), watch for *dilatation lag*, a unilateral slowness of pupil enlargement after the light has been moved away.
- *Test the consensual response.* While shining a torch in one eye, observe the response in the other. If there is no pupillary constriction in either eye in response to light shone in one eye, but normal bilateral constriction in

response to light in the other eye, then there is a *total afferent pupillary defect* of the affected side (*amaurotic pupil*).

- *Intact direct and consensual responses* suggest that both 3rd nerves are functioning, as are both optic nerves; however, it is possible that the function of the optic nerves is asymmetrical. (For example, although still functioning, the right optic nerve may not be functioning as well as the left, as in optic neuritis). Therefore, test for a *relative afferent pupillary defect* (RAPD).

- *Testing for RAPD* (Fig. 28.1). Swing the torch from one eye to the other, allowing at least three seconds of illumination in each eye before returning to the other. As the torch is briskly (important) swung from the healthy eye (both pupils appropriately constricted) to the diseased eye (poorly functioning optic nerve or retina), both pupils will dilate. This represents poorer conduction of impulses in the optic nerve of the affected eye than in the healthy eye and is a vital sign in clinical ophthalmology. Due to the variation between individuals in the amount of pupillary constriction in response to light, an RAPD examination is extremely useful, as it produces an objective result, comparing normal and abnormal within an individual. *Please note that the pupillary responses in an RAPD are bilateral.*

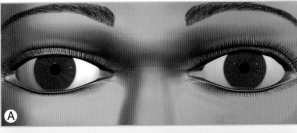
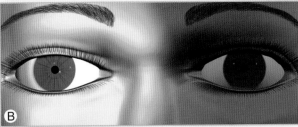
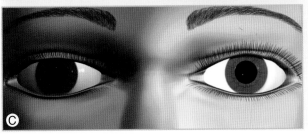

Fig. 28.1 Testing for RAPD. A. A patient with an optic nerve lesion in one eye will not have anisocoria. Thus, in this patient with a left optic nerve lesion, both pupils are equal. **B.** If a bright light is shone into the normal eye (right), both pupils will constrict; this also shows that both efferent responses (pupil constriction) are normal in this case. **C.** If the light is shone into the affected eye (left), both pupils will dilate, as there is a reduced afferent conduction of nerve impulses in the diseased optic nerve.

Further Information

Grading of RAPDs

RAPDs can be graded using *neutral density filters*. A neutral density filter is placed before the healthy eye and an RAPD examination performed. If there is still a relative difference in pupillary constriction (in both eyes) despite the filter, denser filters are selected until no difference exists between the two eyes. The final neutral density filter selected represents the severity of the RAPD, i.e. the amount of 'dulling' of the light in the good eye needed to make the two eyes' responses equal. This measurement can then be repeated to compare the severity of the optic nerve lesion with time.

- *In the presence of an objective RAPD*, it is also possible to elicit a subjective RAPD, which may add more weight to a clinical diagnosis if the signs are subtle. While shining the light in the healthy eye, ask the patient to compare the brightness of the light as it moves to the affected eye (e.g. 'If the light here in the good eye is ten out of ten, how much is the other eye?' 'Two out of ten, doctor.').

- *Now check the accommodative responses.* Turn the room lights on again. Compare the size of the pupils when fixating a distant target and then when fixating a near target. It is important that the near target is an accommodative stimulus (such as a toy or figure) rather than a non-accommodative target such as a torch, in order to stimulate the pupillary near reflex. It is best to hold the near target almost in line with the distant target, so that changing fixation is not accompanied by large saccades. *Light-near dissociation* is the absence of pupillary constriction with light, but preserved pupillary constriction for accommodation.

- *Slitlamp examination.* Examine for segmental vermiform movements ('like a worm') of the iris, which represent the response to light in the face of partial denervation of the sphincter pupillae (tonic pupil). Look for evidence of traumatic mydriasis, such as iris sphincter rupture, and the presence of pseudophakia. Some patients who have received a corneal graft may also have a fixed mydriasis.

- *Consider checking the eye movements.* If there is an efferent defect (3rd nerve), consider whether there may be associated oculomotor defects or evidence of aberrant regeneration.

- *General examination if needed.* Tendon reflexes may be depressed in the Holmes–Adie syndrome. Argyll Robertson pupils are bilaterally small and irregular, and exhibit light-near dissociation. There may be many other signs of associated systemic disease, as encountered in associated diabetes mellitus or syphilis. A full neurological examination is recommended if cranial nerve lesions are present.

29

Cover testing

JP Kersey

Introduction

Large squints are easily seen from a distance, but smaller squints (e.g. < 10 prism dioptres (Δ)) can be easily missed. The different kinds of cover testing identify all squints and also allow their differentiation into manifest squints (*heterotropias* or *tropias*) or latent squints (*heterophorias* or *phorias*, a tendency to squint), as well as their subsequent measurement.

It is important during the initial part of a cover test examination not to *dissociate* a patient, as this will uncover a latent component of the squint, which the patient may not be able to easily recover from.

Cover/uncover test

The cover/uncover test (Fig. 29.1) is performed to detect a squint. The movement of each eye in turn is observed, as first the left and then the right eye is covered and then uncovered. The test should be performed both with and without spectacles, and with and without any compensatory head posture that the patient may have adopted.

- The patient is asked to fixate on a distant target (usually at 6 m).
- The first eye is covered (e.g. the left). The right eye is then observed to see whether it moves to take up fixation. If it does so, this implies that the right eye was not looking at the same target as the left eye prior to being covered (and therefore a squint must be present). If the eye moves outwards to take up fixation, then a convergent squint (*esotropia*) is present. If the eye moves inwards, then a divergent squint (*exotropia*) is present.
- The left eye is then uncovered and the movement of the right eye is observed. If the left eye again takes up fixation, a movement will be made by the right eye, outwards for an exotropia or inwards for an esotropia.
- The test is then repeated for the other eye.
- If when performing a cover test on the left eye, no movement of the right eye is noticed, but when cover testing the right eye, the left eye moves to take up fixation, this would be known as a left tropia (esotropia or exotropia). The converse is true for right tropias (where left eye fixation is preferred).
- The test is then repeated using a near accommodative target (e.g. mini-Snellen chart or small attention-holding picture on a stick at one third of a metre/33 cm). The use of a near target activates the 'near response', the triad of convergence, miosis and accommodation. Some patients have a different

Examination of patients

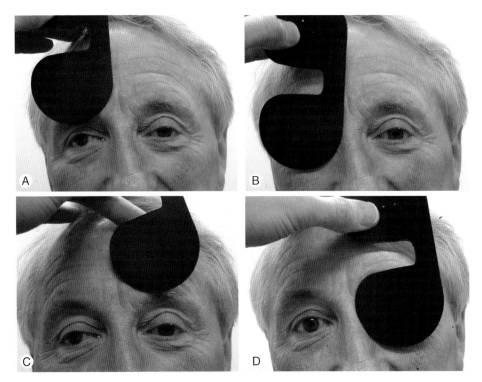

Fig. 29.1 Example of a cover/uncover test. A. This patient with a right divergent squint is fixating with his left eye. **B.** Covering the squinting right eye causes no movement of the left eye. **C.** Prior to covering the left eye, fixation is still with the left eye. **D.** Covering the left eye causes a medial movement of the right eye to take up fixation, proving that the right eye had definitely been squinting.

squint for near and distance, which is often (but not always) due to abnormal or excessive convergence induced as part of accommodation. Thus, although there may be no squint seen in a distance cover test, there may well be a squint on a near cover test.

The cover/uncover test also works for vertical deviations, when an initial upward movement of the eye not being covered indicates a *hypodeviation* in that eye, while a downwards movement indicates a *hyperdeviation*.

Alternate cover test

This is a *dissociative* test and aims to identify the sum of both the manifest and latent components of the squint.

- One eye (e.g. the left) is covered while the patient is asked to look at a distant (6 m) target.
- The occluder is then quickly moved over to the other eye. The movement of the eye which was uncovered is carefully observed to see how far it needs to

move to take up fixation. A lateral movement indicates an *esodeviation*, while a medial movement indicates an *exodeviation*.

- If no squint was evident on the original cover/uncover test, these movements are known as either an *esophoria* or an *exophoria* (latent deviations), or if a squint was previously seen, the deviation seen is the sum of the latent and manifest parts of the squint (usually more than the original squint alone).

- The amount of latent deviation seen may increase with time as the test continues (and the eyes become more and more dissociated).

- This test is then repeated at $\frac{1}{3}$ m.

- Information regarding the relative visual acuity of each eye can occasionally be gleaned from the cover tests by observing the speed with which each eye takes up fixation. If one eye is very slow (sometimes requiring encouragement!), it is certainly possible that there is poor acuity in that eye.

Prism cover test

This test allows the measurement of the angle of deviation, which provides quantification and documentation of the squint. This allows monitoring of the progression of the squint with time and allows the planning of surgery.

A prism is held in front of the deviating eye in manifest squints (tropias) and before either eye in latent deviations (phorias).

- The patient is asked to fixate a 6 m target.

- An alternate cover test is performed.

- If the uncovered eye moves medially (exodeviation), a base-in prism is needed to correct the movement. If a lateral movement is seen (esodeviation), a base-out prism is needed.

- The alternate cover test is then repeated with a prism in place and if a further movement is seen, the prism is then altered. If the movement is in the same direction, then the prism strength needs to be increased; if the movement has reversed, then the prism strength needs to be reduced.

- This is repeated until no movement is seen. In combined horizontal and vertical deviations, a combination of vertical and horizontal prisms may be needed.

- The size of the prism required is noted and the test is then repeated in other positions of gaze (preferably the nine diagnostic positions of gaze).

- The test is then also repeated with a $\frac{1}{3}$ m target (although usually just in the primary position).

- For information on how to document the results of prism cover tests and other orthoptic tests, see Appendix 1.

Prism reflection test

If the patient is unable to cooperate with a formal prism cover test, then corneal reflections can be used to identify a deviation and prisms can be placed in front of one eye and altered until the reflections are equal.

Examination of patients

Hirschberg's test

A rough estimate of a deviation can be gained using Hirschberg's test.

- A torch is shone at the squinting patient, which produces dissimilar corneal reflections.
- The fixing eye will have a central reflection while the non-fixing eye will have a deviated reflection.
- If the reflection in the non-fixing eye is at the pupil margin, this approximates to a 15° (or 30 Δ) deviation, a reflection at the limbus approximates to a 45° (or 90 Δ) deviation, and a reflection halfway between the pupil and limbus approximates to a 25° (or 50 Δ) deviation.

All of these tests (and many others) are routinely performed by orthoptists. They are the best source of expertise to observe and advise on technique.

Occluders

Most occluders are totally opaque, usually black pieces of plastic. This means that it is impossible to see what the covered eye is doing during the cover test— it can only be inferred as to what happened by watching the eye's recovery movements after removing the occluder.

Some occluders (e.g. the Spielmann), which are sadly often prohibitively expensive, are not totally opaque, but are sufficiently so to cause dissociation of the eyes. Through the use of such an occluder, unusual movements of the covered eye (e.g. dissociated vertical deviation) can also be seen during the cover tests.

Examination of eye movements

JP Kersey

Introduction

The proper examination of eye movements requires a lot of practice and a good routine. The following is designed as a suggested routine that will also double as a checklist for Examinations.

There are many parts to this examination and a degree of discretion needs to be used to decide whether certain parts are relevant.

Suggested routine

- Introduction to the patient.
- Look carefully at the patient. Are there any signs of:
  - abnormal head posture (adopted to maintain binocular single vision)
  - proptosis
  - scars, plombs (used in retinal detachment surgery)
  - ptosis, lid retraction
  - dilated pupils
  - redness over the conjunctiva
  - strabismus
  - prosthesis
  - systemic signs of weakness, e.g. a wheelchair.
- Ask to check the visual acuity, check to see if the patient is wearing glasses (highly myopic?) and if so whether there is evidence of a Fresnel prism on them.
- Perform a cover test (Ch. 29) in the *primary position* (looking straight ahead), which should be done for both near and distance, with and without glasses. Ideally, this should also be performed both with and without any abnormal compensatory head posture. This step is often skipped in an Examination (at the Examiners' request!).
- Next remove the glasses and use a bright torch to examine the corneal reflexes. An estimate of the deviation can be made using Hirschberg's test (Ch. 29).

Examination of patients

- Ask the patient how many lights are seen (one or two) and to let you know if they see double during the examination.

- Establish if the patient has any pain on eye movement. Ask the patient to follow the torch as you move it into the *secondary positions* of gaze (horizontal and vertical positions). Binocular movements of the eyes are called *versions*, as opposed to *ductions*, which are uniocular movements.

- Check for differences in lid height such as:

  - narrowing in adduction, seen in Duane's syndrome

  - widening in adduction, seen in aberrant 3rd nerve regeneration

  - look for differences in pupil size during eye movements (aberrant regeneration).

- Move the torch into the *tertiary positions* of gaze (oblique positions or diagonals).

- If diplopia is seen in any of the positions, ask whether it is horizontal, vertical or torsional. Find out which position of gaze it is greatest in and check which image disappears upon covering one of the eyes. In the lateral positions of gaze, the more peripheral image comes from the more paretic eye (this is known as 'analysing' or 'mapping' the diplopia).

- Uniocular eye movements (ductions) can be tested if a limitation is noted in one of the eyes during versions. To do this, cover the eye that seems to be moving normally and repeat the examination—does the limitation decrease?

Further Information

Ductions and versions

If the duction movement is greater than the version movement, this implies a neurogenic cause. A restrictive cause will produce ductions and versions of similar magnitude.

- If there is any difference in height between the two eyes in the primary position, consider performing a cover test in left and right gaze, followed by left and right head tilt (Bielchowsky head tilt). This sequence is termed Parks' three-step test, which is often used in clinical practice to diagnose 4th nerve palsies (see box at end of chapter).

- Comment on whether the smooth pursuit movements are normal or jerky. Also comment on the presence of any nystagmus and then describe it.

- *Nystagmus.* This is described initially by the direction of the fast phase and can help to identify the site of the lesion, e.g. upbeat/downbeat, left beat/right beat. Secondly, what makes the nystagmus worse? Gaze-induced nystagmus is worse on looking to extremes of gaze. Is there a null point? In other words, is there a position of the eyes where the nystagmus is reduced? There are also rarer variations of nystagmus, including rotational, opsiclonus, convergence-retraction and alternating. These are well-described elsewhere in more clinical texts.

- Next test the saccades. This is done using two targets, e.g. a torch and a finger. Ask the patient to 'look at my torch and then at my finger'. One target should be in the primary position while the other is in one of the secondary positions of gaze. Start with the horizontal positions and then move onto the vertical. Patients should be instructed not to move the head during testing and to attempt not to blink between eye movements (common). Saccades are slow in conditions such as Parkinson's disease, internuclear ophthalmoplegia and myasthenia gravis, and are increased in cerebellar disease. They may also be abnormal in gaze palsies.

- Test vergence. This will help differentiate between a muscle weakness and a gaze palsy, as the neuronal pathway for vergence is different to that of versions. Test this using an accommodative target from about 30 cm away and bring it towards the patient to about 10 cm. The pupils should also constrict, confirming the convergence pathway is being activated.

- Other tests can allow differentiation between peripheral (muscle or nerve lesions) and central (gaze or supranuclear palsies) lesions. If these tests are normal, but the patient is unable to look in a particular direction on demand, it is possible that there is a supranuclear (or functional) disorder of eye movement, as intact reflexes imply satisfactorily functioning extraocular muscles. This is a difficult clinical area and the junior ophthalmologist should probably consult with a senior at this stage.

  - *Optokinetic nystagmus* (OKN). This uses a rotating striped drum, which is rotated initially horizontally and then vertically to induce a nystagmus. The vertical component is good at detecting convergence retraction nystagmus, as seen when rotating the drum downwards in Parinaud's syndrome of the midbrain.

  - *Vestibular-ocular reflex* (VOR). This is tested by asking the patient to read the Snellen chart while making small head-nodding movements.

  - *Doll's head movements* (also tests VOR, but generally used in less compliant patients, e.g. intensive care patients).

- Consider testing:

  - Pupillary examination: will be needed if a 3rd nerve palsy is suspected.

  - Lid fatigability should be tested to exclude myasthenia. This is done by measuring the palpebral aperture then asking the patient to look up for 60 seconds and then re-measuring the aperture. If the levator muscle is fatigued, the lid will drop.

  - Cogan's lid twitch: an overshoot of the eyelid as the patient makes a saccade from below to the primary position—sometimes seen in myasthenia.

- Further investigation may include:

  - Hess test (see Ch. 36).

  - Visual field testing.

  - Imaging of the brain, especially the nerve pathways of the 3rd, 4th and 6th cranial nerves.

Examination of patients

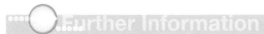

Further Information

Parks' three-step test

This test is used to identify the weak muscle when vertical diplopia is present (usually a superior oblique). It relies on an understanding of the positions of gaze in which the four vertically-acting muscles (i.e. all but the horizontal recti) are strongest. The superior and inferior recti are strongest on lateral gaze, where they elevate and depress the eye, respectively. Likewise, adducting the eye places the superior and inferior obliques in their optimum positions for depressing or elevating the eye, respectively. Careful analysis of the eyes in different positions of gaze should allow the clinician to work out which muscle is under-acting. This careful analysis is done by cover testing and watching the vertical movements of the eyes in different positions of gaze, with each step of the test reducing the number of possibilities for the under-acting muscle by half. It should be stated that this test only produces useful results if only one muscle is affected.

For example, consider the three-step test in a patient complaining of new-onset vertical diplopia.

- *Step 1.* Cover testing in the primary position shows the right eye is higher than the left; this can be thought of as either a right hypertropia or a left hypotropia. This suggests that either the inferior rectus or superior oblique in the right eye is at fault, meaning the right eye is not being pulled down enough, OR the superior rectus or inferior oblique in the left eye is at fault, meaning the left eye is not being pulled up enough.

- *Step 2.* Cover testing in both right and left gaze shows the right hypertropia is worse in left gaze (remember: left gaze is produced by combination of right adduction and left abduction). If the weak muscle is a right eye muscle, it is the right superior oblique not pulling the eye down enough; if it is a left eye muscle that is weak, it is the left superior rectus not pulling the eye up enough. This reduces the number of possibilities for the under-acting muscle to two. Distinguishing these two is done with the Bielchowsky head tilt.

- *Step 3.* Cover testing in presence of head tilt to both right and left reveals that the right hypertropia is worse on tilting the head to the right. The muscles with the prefix 'superior' both intort the eye, whereas the inferior muscles extort the eye. To compensate for a head tilt to the right, the right eye must intort and the left eye extort. The worsening of the hypertropia on right tilt implies that the right eye is unable to intort and the superior rectus is overacting to compensate, so increasing the height of that eye. In view of this and the results of steps 1 and 2, the right superior oblique is therefore at fault.

Remembering the actions of these muscles may be made easier with the following mnemonic: RADSIN – Recti ADduct, Superior INtort.

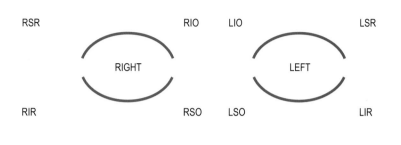

RSR   RIO   LIO   LSR

RIGHT   LEFT

RIR   RSO   LSO   LIR

Fig. 30.1 Diagram showing the optimum positions for testing the different vertically acting muscles. Remember these are *not* the directions of actions of the muscles.

31

Examination of the orbit

SN Madge

Introduction

Although possible, you are unlikely to be asked to 'examine the orbit' in an Examination because it would take far too long to be done properly. Nevertheless, there are a multitude of clinical conditions where a comprehensive orbital examination is required, for example thyroid eye disease, trauma and tumours.

Below is a suggested scheme for orbital examination. Where appropriate, the reader is suggested to consult the relevant chapters of the book for information on testing pupil reactions, visual fields, etc.

Suggested routine

- Introduction to patient.
- Look carefully at the patient. Are there any obvious signs of:
  - proptosis or enophthalmos
  - a prosthetic eye
  - obvious masses
  - obvious globe pulsation
  - strabismus and dystopia
  - scars
  - pupillary abnormalities
  - ptosis or lid retraction
  - skin capillary haemangiomata
  - periorbital swelling/oedema
  - thyrotoxicosis, e.g. sweating, tremor, agitated state, pretibial myxoedema
  - other abnormal appearances, e.g. Paget's disease, cachexia of malignancy, acromegaly, neurofibromatosis, etc.
- Establish whether the patient is in any pain.
- Check the visual acuity (Ch. 25). Note at this stage whether the patient is wearing spectacles, and if so, are there prisms (Fresnel or otherwise) incorporated? Highly myopic patients may experience mechanical limitation of eye movements.

- Check colour vision (Ch. 22). Abnormalities may represent an early sign of optic nerve compression.

- Check the visual fields by confrontation (Ch. 26). If abnormal, consider formal documentation of the fields by either the Goldmann method (preferred) or automated perimetry (Ch. 23).

- Check sensation in the sensory areas supplied by nerves emanating from the orbit, paying special attention to the infraorbital nerve in cases of trauma (may imply inferior 'blow-out' fracture).

- Perform a cover test and check the eye movements (Chs 29 and 30). Note specifically whether there is any pain on movement, diplopia and restriction of movement (as opposed to a neurogenic palsy). If restriction is suspected, this could be further investigated with a Hess test (Ch. 36) and confirmed with a forced duction test. Restricted movements are often followed over time by plotting uniocular fields of fixation (using the Goldmann apparatus). Check Bell's phenomenon in the presence of obvious proptosis.

- Check for proptosis and enophthalmos with the Hertel exophthalmometer (Ch. 18). If all appears normal at this stage, or in the presence of a skin capillary haemangioma, consider performing exophthalmometry with the Valsalva manoeuvre, and also comparing the results in the sitting and lying positions. Significant differences may indicate pathology such as orbital varices and orbital haemangiomata.

- Check the pupillary responses, looking in particular for a relative afferent pupillary defect (Ch. 28).

- Palpate the orbital rim, feeling for masses. Check the regional lymph nodes (in the event of previous skin tumour spread—should be scars).

- Examine the anterior segment of the eyes at the slitlamp (Chs 32 and 33), in particular looking for:

  - Chemosis and conjunctival hyperaemia, especially over the insertion of the recti.

  - Subconjunctival haemorrhage or emphysema, especially if no posterior limit visible (may suggest orbital 'blow-out' fracture).

  - Signs of corneal exposure.

  - Superior limbic keratoconjunctivitis (associated with thyroid eye disease).

  - Lagophthalmos.

  - Lacrimal gland masses (associated with 'S'-shaped lid contour).

  - Intraocular pressure (in primary position and also with patient looking in direction of restriction of movement; will lead to IOP increase if restricted—rather than paretic—muscle). Also check for pulsation—may be more marked than normal in vascular conditions, e.g. caroticocavernous fistula.

- Examine the posterior segment of the eyes at the slitlamp (Chs 32 and 33), in particular looking for:

  - Optic disc abnormalities, in particular: optic atrophy, optociliary shunt vessels and swelling of the disc. Spontaneous pulsation of the retinal vein is a reassuring sign.

  - Choroidal folds: associated with any orbital mass.

- Retinal vascular abnormalities, such as central retinal vein occlusion or isolated venous dilatation (may imply raised orbital venous pressure), vascular occlusions, etc.

- Metastatic disease.

- Finally, consider listening for a bruit if a caroticocavernous fistula is suspected. Listen with the bell of the stethoscope. Is the bruit diminished with ipsilateral carotid compression (take care to avoid precipitating syncope)?

- Retropulsion of the globe (i.e. pushing the globe posteriorly with the pulp of a finger) often provides useful information to experienced clinicians about the nature of proptosis. It is not recommended in the setting of an Examination as it may cause pain.

- Ancillary investigations include:

  - Imaging of the orbit: CT scanning is better at delineating bony abnormalities, while MRI scanning is better for soft tissue abnormalities. However, local protocol will usually dictate.

  - Plain X-rays of the orbit often suffice in the setting of suspected orbital 'blow-out' fractures, provided that no abnormalities of ocular movements or optic nerve function are noted. Also ensure that there is no concurrent fracture of the zygoma on the X-ray (common, needs maxillofacial intervention soon).

  - Functional tests of optic nerve function, including visual evoked potentials (often used in the monitoring of patients with thyroid eye disease).

  - Tests of ocular motility, including the Hess test (Ch. 36) and field of uniocular (and binocular single) vision.

  - Systemic investigations where appropriate, e.g. thyroid function test and chest radiograph.

32

Examination of the anterior segment with the slitlamp

SN Madge

Introduction

Use of the slitlamp is a fundamental skill for all ophthalmic practitioners. Its various controls are described elsewhere (Ch. 12), and this chapter focuses on the appropriate clinical use of the machine. What follows is a suggested routine for examining the anterior segment of the eye, which will allow all relevant clinical signs to be appreciated without missing some more subtle, but important (especially in Examinations) findings.

General remarks

Do not move the slitlamp rapidly, as this can make patients very nervous and can potentially damage the equipment. Ensure that the patient is comfortable prior to the start of the examination, as this will make subsequent steps much easier.

Preparation

- Give a clear introduction to the patient and explain what you will be doing.
- Before asking the patient to move to the chin rest, check the machine thoroughly and ensure that:
    - The height of the machine, the patient and yourself are all similar.
    - The eyepieces are completely pushed into their sockets and that the focus for each is correct for your own desired settings.
    - You are familiar with the controls of the particular model of slitlamp you are using.
    - The wall power supply is on (!).
    - The slitlamp is not currently aligned for sclerotic scatter—if so, tighten the appropriate knob (Ch. 12).
    - The magnification and brightness settings are what you are expecting.
    - The table-top brake is off.
    - The floor-brake (if appropriate) is on.
- Having already estimated the correct height of the machine relative to the patient, adjust the height of the chin rest. Ask the patient to move to the chin rest and to place the forehead firmly against the upper bar. Check that the

height is comfortable for the patient and ensure that the lateral orbital rim is aligned with the black mark on the adjacent frame. If not, ask the patient to move back off the bar before adjusting the height again.

- Turn the power switch on and make a slow approach to the right eye.

Examination

- Using the ×10 power, coaxial illumination and grey-filtered light (to reduce glare and also allowing the patient to get used to the bright light), take a low-powered view of the eye, eyelids and their margins. Are there any obvious abnormalities? While retracting the relevant eyelid, ask the patient to look up, down, left and right. Trabeculectomy blebs, symblepharon, pinguecula, conjunctival scarring and corneal lesions otherwise hidden by the eyelids will all become obvious. Are there any obvious abnormalities of the conjunctiva, cornea, lens, iris or pupil? Note the iris colour (of each eye).

- Increase the power to ×16, remove the grey filter and rotate the illumination column to the side of the eye being examined. Ask the patient to fixate your contralateral ear.

- Examine in turn:

  - The corneal epithelium, stroma and endothelium, ensuring that cornea covered by the lids is not neglected. If necessary, perform sclerotic scatter and specular microscopy (see below).

  - The anterior chamber, looking for chamber depth, cells and flare. Set the slit beam to 3 mm height and 1 mm width and look for the above in the obliquely passing beam (like watching dust float in a cinema beam).

  - The lens or intraocular lens implant (IOL). Oblique illumination allows assessment of nuclear sclerosis; coaxial illumination will allow posterior subcapsular opacities (cataract) and posterior capsular opacities (IOL) to be easily detected.

  - The iris. In particular, ensure that retroillumination is performed: reduce the height and width of the slitlamp to 1 mm and using unfiltered, coaxial light through the centre of the pupil, look to see if the red reflex is visible through the iris ('transillumination defects'). Ensure that all of the iris is visible at the time by manually retracting the lids if necessary. Superior laser peripheral iridotomies will soon become obvious. Note the presence or absence of pseudoexfoliative matter that may only be obvious on the iris margin in an undilated patient.

  - The anterior vitreous, if possible. With an undilated pupil, pass unfiltered light in a 1 mm by 1 mm beam obliquely through the pupil. Tobacco dust or inflammatory cells may be obvious. Examination of the vitreous is, of course, better done with a dilated pupil.

- Move to examine the other eye slowly. Start, as above, from a distance. In particular, note immediately any difference in iris colour and pupillary movement.

- To complete the examination, evert both upper lids and measure the intraocular pressure (see 'Tonometry', Ch. 34) (probably neither in Examinations, but offer). Offer to examine the posterior segment (see 'Retinal examination at the slitlamp', Ch. 33). Consider using fluorescein and re-examining the anterior segment, including performing the Seidel test (see below).

- Ask the patient to relax back off the machine and turn it off.
- For information on how to document your findings, see Appendix 1.

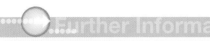

Sclerotic scatter

Having uncoupled the microscope from the illumination column (Ch. 12), shine the light beam on the limbus while focusing on the corneal area of interest. Total internal reflection of light through the cornea allows stromal opacities to become more obvious than under direct illumination alone.

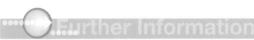

Specular microscopy

This is a uniocular technique, which is useful for examining the corneal endothelium and anterior lens capsule. The best images are often obtained with the use of a contact lens and high magnification; if possible, change the ×10 eyepieces to the ×16 eyepieces. Using the protractor scale at the common hinge, align the illumination column and microscope so that the patient's gaze bisects the angle between the two (e.g. 30° between microscope and patient, and patient and illumination). Using unfiltered light, focus on the structure of interest *monocularly*. A *specular* reflection should be visible, although there may be a great deal of glare visible immediately adjacent to the structure. Careful focusing should allow individual endothelial cells (for example) to be seen.

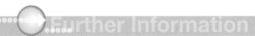

Fluorescein and the Seidel test

The anionic substance fluorescein has the useful property of emitting a yellow–green colour when blue light is shone upon it (fluorescence). It also stains epithelial defects and is therefore very useful in examining the anterior cornea, especially if one is inexperienced. Additional topical anaesthesia is not required. The Seidel test reveals any leaks of aqueous from the eye, e.g. in the setting of suspected globe rupture or a poorly-constructed surgical incision. Fluorescein 2% is applied and blue light shone on the eye. If there is an aqueous leak, a clear 'river' of non-fluorescing fluid (aqueous) may be seen running (typically with gravity) through the fluorescing, yellow/green, surrounding fluorescein.

Retinal examination at the slitlamp

SN Madge

Introduction

Please ensure that you are familiar with all the controls of the slitlamp and are capable of a basic slitlamp anterior segment examination prior to attempting retinal examination with one of the many available lenses (Chs 12 and 32).

Principles

The overall optical power of the eye (≈58 D) is such that only relatively anterior structures can be seen with the slitlamp. In order to see the more posterior structures including the retina, either a strong *plus* lens (e.g. +90 D, producing an optically real but inverted image) or a strong *minus* lens (e.g. Hruby lens, producing an optically virtual but upright image) must be used.

The Hruby lens is now very rarely used; the image quality is poor and was very susceptible to patient movement (in comparison to the real images seen with convex lenses). They are often to be found attached to a metal pole in the drawer of slitlamp tables which attaches to the patient examination frame.

In more common use these days are the convex lenses, with the common types being the +90 D, +78 D and +66 D (differences discussed in brief below). A real image of the retina is formed between the lens and the slitlamp, which is then magnified by the lenses incorporated into the slitlamp.

Some contact lenses can also be used to view the retina while at the slitlamp. For example, the central window of the beloved Goldmann three-mirror lens acts as a powerful concave lens, forming a virtual, non-inverted image of the retina. Many clinics will also have dedicated 'macular lenses', which provide an excellent stereoscopic view of the posterior pole and are the gold standard for clinical detection of retinal thickening. Other lenses, often used in laser photocoagulation treatments, generally provide an inverted real image of the retina. For information on how to apply contact lenses to the eye, see Chapter 17 ('Gonioscopy and three-mirror examination'); then proceed as below to obtain an image, bearing in mind whether your image will be inverted or not.

How to do it

Only non-contact convex lenses (e.g. of the +90 D type) are discussed in this chapter. For such lenses, remember you will be observing an inverted view of the retina.

- Select the appropriate light source (usually best to start with the grey filter in place) and size (e.g. 8 mm vertical slit and 1–1.5 mm width). (Always ensure that the heat filter is in place if not using the grey filter.)
- Ask the patient to fixate your ear (right ear for examining the patient's right eye and vice versa) and align the slitlamp with the centre of the pupil.
- Pull the slitlamp approximately two-thirds of the way back from its anterior segment focus position.
- Holding the lens between thumb and forefinger, place at least one of your spare fingers on the patient's forehead to steady yourself. Keeping the lens perpendicular to the axis between the patient's eyes and the lenses of the slitlamp, place the lens about 1 cm from the patient's eye (Fig. 33.1).
- If one side of the lens is coloured white (on its rim), then place this side closest to the patient; this provides the least optical aberrations if using an aspheric lens.
- If a beginner, have a quick look around the side of the slitlamp to ensure that your lens is held at the correct level—a common mistake is to let the lens drift downwards producing a highly magnified, inverted view of the patient's nose instead! An experienced observer, by watching the light reflexes entering the eye, can assist in helping you find an image.
- An orange glow (of the retina) should appear. To focus, simply move the joystick back and forth until the inverted image of the retina comes into view. If the patient is fixating your ear, the optic disc should come into view (unless your patient has a squint!).
- Once you have an image, adjust the various light controls to minimise patient discomfort and maximise your view.

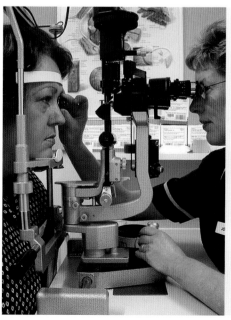

Fig. 33.1 Examination of the retina using a +90 D lens. Note the correct position of the patient on the chin rest, with her forehead against the bar, the lens being held perpendicular to the axis between patient and slitlamp, the lens being held at the same height as the eye and approximately 1 cm from it, and also the position of the slitlamp on the tabletop (approximately ²⁄₃ of the available travel back).

- To look to the left, keep the lens still initially and move the joystick to the left (remembering that the you are actually looking to the retina to your right, as the image is inverted). Similarly, to go up, keep the lens still and rotate the joystick clockwise (remembering that more inferior retina is coming into view, as the image is inverted).

- To examine more peripheral retina, ask the patient to look in the required direction, re-centre the light reflex over the obliquely looking pupil and try again. To start with, keep the lens perpendicular to the patient–slitlamp axis, but you will soon find that the image improves with a little tilting for examining the periphery.

- Some more advanced Haag–Streit slitlamps may be equipped with a stereo-variator device, which enhances the posterior segment stereoscopic field of view and may aid the examination of: highly myopic fundi; fundi in the presence of small pupils; and also the peripheral vitreous and fundus. If present on the slitlamp, there will be an additional dial on the microscope body, usually in front of the rotating bank of lenses. Rotate the dial through 90°, offset the illumination column by a few degrees (usually clicks into place) and try using the 90 D. If left in place for anterior segment examination, the stereo-variator will give greatly reduced stereopsis, making anterior chambers look very shallow.

Other lenses (Fig. 33.2)

- A +90 D lens gives a wide field of view but has limited magnification. It is therefore very good for examining large areas of the retina quickly, but less useful for detailed examination of the optic disc or macula.

- In contrast, the +66 D lens provides excellent magnification but has a much more limited field of view; it is therefore ideal for examination of the macula and optic disc, but less useful for examining the peripheral retina.

- The +78 D lens provides a halfway house option between the two other lenses.

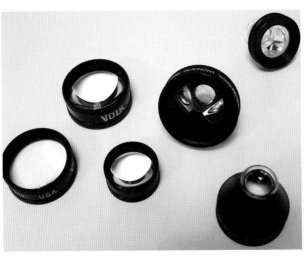

Fig. 33.2 Some of the many lenses used in the examination of the retina.

- In general, the higher the power of the lens, the easier is the view through an undilated pupil; thus in a glaucoma clinic, although it would be desirable to view all optic discs with a +66 D lens (ideal for measuring disc size, see below), it is nigh on impossible unless the pupil is dilated and therefore a +90 D lens is often substituted.

- Other non-contact fundus lenses exist with variable characteristics.

- The slitlamp needs to be focused further away from the patient with a +66 D than with a +90 D.

- The +66 D lens has a relative magnification of approximately 1.0, which means that it can be used with relative ease to measure the size of, for example, the optic disc, without having to use a correction factor (necessary for the other lenses). By aligning the length of the slitlamp slit with the retinal structure in question, a reading can be read off the scale in millimetres for the size of such structures.

Ametropia

In myopes, the retinal image will increase in size with movement of the lens away from the patient and decrease in size with motion towards the patient. The converse is true in hypermetropia.

Tonometry

R Sidebottom

One of the first completely new skills that the new ophthalmic practitioner must master is measurement of the intraocular pressure (IOP).

Principles

Most tonometers give an indirect measure of IOP using the Imbert–Fick principle, which states that the pressure (P) inside an idealised sphere is equal to the force (F) necessary to flatten the surface divided by the area (A) of flattening (P = F/A). The eye is not an idealised sphere, primarily because corneal rigidity resists the force and the capillary action of the tear film attracts the tonometer prism. The design of the Goldmann tonometer exploits these two opposing forces, as they approximately cancel each other when the applanated area is of 3.06 mm diameter (the diameter of the tonometer prism).

Goldmann applanation tonometer

How to use it (Fig. 34.1)

- Remove the tonometer prism from the disinfectant solution (some units use alcohol wipes), rinse and dry it.
- Insert the prism into the tonometer bracket holder, ensuring the 0° or 180° markings line up with the white line on the bracket. The tonometer is then placed on the slitlamp guide plate and locked there by inserting the peg under the tonometer into one of the holes on the plate. Some tonometers are mounted on a pivot permanently on the slitlamp; to move these into position swing them round until they locate centrally in the measuring position.
- Increase the light source to maximum intensity with the blue filter in place and the slit opened fully. It should illuminate the prism from the side at about 60°. If despite maximum power the tonometer head is not well-lit, then extra light can occasionally be found by uncoupling the slitlamp illumination column from the microscope (Ch. 12).
- Instil a drop of anaesthetic/fluorescein mixture into the eyes. Alternatively, separate local anaesthetic drops and a fluorescein strip may be used.
- Positioning and cooperation of the patient are vital. Ensure the patient is comfortable with the chin on the chin rest and forehead firmly against the bar. Ask the patient to look straight ahead with eyes wide open (say 'stare' rather than 'don't blink').

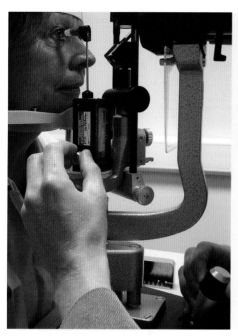

Fig. 34.1 Goldmann tonometry: the approach. Note that the prism and patient are at the same height and that the slitlamp joystick is pointing backwards, ready to carefully place the prism on to the cornea using a fine movement.

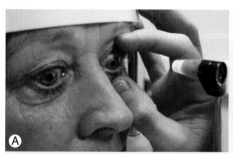
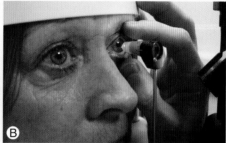

Ⓐ Ⓑ

Fig. 34.2 Holding open the lids in Goldmann tonometry. Carefully holding the lids against the orbital rims allows correct measurement of pressure in patients who are otherwise unable to keep eyes open.

- Patients are often unable to keep the eyes open without blinking, in which case you must gently hold open the lids with one hand (Fig. 34.2). It is important not to apply any pressure to the globe, as this would increase the measured IOP. To avoid this, hold the lids against the orbital rim.

- Advance the whole slitlamp towards the eye with the joystick held towards you (Fig. 34.1). When the tip is within a centimetre or so of the cornea, use the joystick to gently bring the tip into contact under direct vision. The limbus will light up when you have made contact. Ensure the upper lid lashes are avoided, as touching these often stimulates a blink.

Examination of patients

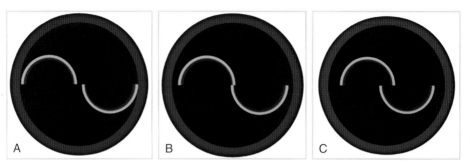

Fig. 34.3 Views down the eyepiece using Goldmann tonometry. A. The rings of fluorescein are too wide apart and the pressure will be measured low. **B.** Rings just touching. Correct reading. **C.** Rings overlap. Pressure will be measured high.

- Look down the slitlamp eyepiece (only one eyepiece will be lined up with the prism). You should see two semicircles of fluorescein shifted away from each other along the horizontal axis (Fig. 34.3).
- Use the slitlamp joystick to position the semicircles at the centre of the prism. Now adjust the dial to alter the force on the prism and thus alter the size and overlap of the semicircles. The end point is when the inner edges are just touching. The overlap will usually vary with ocular pulsation; the correct value is the mid-point of this variation. The intraocular pressure in mmHg is the value on the dial multiplied by ten.

Pitfalls

- If the slitlamp is moved too far forward, the feeler arm will reach its limit. The result is large overlapping semicircles, which do not pulsate and do not change size when the measuring dial is turned.
- The width of the fluorescein semicircles should be about $\frac{1}{10}$th the diameter of the ring. A thin ring indicates insufficient fluorescein and tear film drying. This will underestimate the pressure. Ask the patient to blink or instil more fluorescein and try again. If there is too much fluorescein in the tear film, or the prism touches the upper lid, a thick ring will be seen, resulting in overestimation of the pressure. Dry the prism and repeat.
- Pressing on the globe whilst holding open the patient's lids, or excessive squeezing of the lids by the patient, will result in artificially raised pressure. Wearing a neck tie may also lead to a falsely raised IOP measurement.
- Corneal anatomy is assumed to be normal; inaccurate values will result from the presence of abnormal corneal thickness or pathology such as distortion. It is possible to measure corneal thickness with a pachymeter and make an approximate correction to the value obtained.
- Repeating the measurement allows you to take an average to improve the accuracy.

Further Information

Patients with marked astigmatism

In patients with astigmatism of greater than 3 D, the applanated area will be elliptical, not circular. This error can be avoided by applanation at 43° to the meridian of the greatest radius or axis of *minus* cylinder (see 'Basic clinical optics' section). This is done by lining up the angle of *minus* cylinder on the prism graduation with the red mark on the prism holder.

Further Information

Calibration of the Goldmann tonometer

It is possible to check the calibration of the tonometer. This is done at dial position 0, 2 and 6 (0, 20 and 60 mmHg equivalents).

- Insert the prism in the holder and place the tonometer on the slitlamp.
- At setting 0, the feeler arm should be in free movement; if the dial position is moved to –0.05 the arm should fall towards the examiner, if the drum is moved to position +0.05 the arm should fall towards the patient.
- To check settings 2 and 6, the check weight is used (this is normally found in the case with the tonometer prisms or in the drawer of the slitlamp). There are five markings engraved on the bar. These represent 0 centrally, then 2 on either side and 6 towards the edges. Line up the adjustable holder with index mark 2 on the weight. With the longer end of the bar facing you, put it into the insert on the side of the tonometer and push all the way in. Repeat the above manoeuvre (for setting 0), this time moving the dial from 2 to 1.95 and 2.05. To check position 6, move the weight bar to the end position and repeat at 6 rotating to 6.1 and 5.9. If these measurements show that the tonometer is inaccurate, it should be returned to the manufacturer for recalibration.

Other types of tonometer

Perkins

The Perkins tonometer works on the same principle as the Goldmann but is portable and does not require a slitlamp, allowing measurement of the supine patient. It is often more difficult to get accurate readings.

Tonopen

The tonopen uses a force transducer and microprocessor to calculate the IOP. It is a self-contained battery powered device useful for children, supine patients and gross corneal pathology. The tonopen is less accurate than a Goldmann, especially at extremes of pressure.

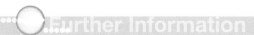

Further Information

How to use the Tonopen

Ensure that there is a new rubber cover over the tip. Instil an anaesthetic drop into the eye. Turn on the tonopen by holding down the button. It will require calibrating on start-up (for a given day); this is done by holding it tip down, then when it displays 'UP' on the readout hold it tip pointing upwards. Repeatedly tap the tonopen gently on the central cornea; it beeps with each reading then gives a longer beep when it has enough results. An average value will be supplied on the readout along with a 5% (best) to >20% confidence value. Do not leave the tonopen without a new rubber cover on the tip (even in its box) as this protects the mechanism from dust.

Non-contact tonometers

These are devices used primarily by optometrists in the community, which use a puff of air to applanate an area of cornea, which is optically sensed by the machine. They are less accurate than Goldmann tonometers and tend to overestimate pressures.

A general approach to ophthalmic problems

SN Madge

Introduction

The eye is a complex organ and there may be many possible causes for loss or reduction in vision. When faced with an anxious patient with visual problems, it is very easy to jump to conclusions that may prejudice your examination and yield incorrect diagnoses. It is important to examine patients in a logical and stepwise manner so that no signs are neglected.

A suggested scheme for examination

For instructions on use of the slitlamp and other examination techniques, please refer to the appropriate chapters. For information on how to document your findings, please refer to Appendix 1.

In general, start at the front of the eye and work backwards. A good example of this technique in action is with the patient who has suffered a traumatic injury to the periorbital region and who is complaining of a reduction in vision. As with any medical examination, consider carefully whether a chaperone is required, particularly if the patient has been drinking excessively (as is often the case with trauma).

- Take a history, particularly concentrating on the type of injury and whether any damage to the globe is likely to be due to blunt or sharp means.
- Check the visual acuity, with spectacles if appropriate, and with a pinhole if subnormal (Ch. 25). Ensure that the visual axis is free from obstruction (i.e. swollen eyelids). Near vision is useful to test if macular pathology is suspected.
- Look for enophthalmos or proptosis, using an exophthalmometer if possible (Ch. 18).
- Check infraorbital nerve sensation bilaterally.
- If possible, check colour vision (optic nerve damage) bilaterally (Ch. 22). Consider checking for red desaturation if optic nerve pathology possible (especially optic neuritis). For red desaturation, ask the patient to compare the colour of a bright red object between the two eyes; in optic neuritis, the affected eye will often see a darker shade of red.
- Check eye movements, examining carefully for diplopia, pain and any restriction of eye movements (Ch. 30).
- Check for a relative afferent pupillary defect (RAPD) and other pupillary abnormalities (Ch. 28).

- If possible, examine the lids and fornices for retained foreign bodies and lacerations.
- Examine the conjunctiva looking carefully for lacerations, possible entry sites, foreign bodies, subconjunctival emphysema and haemorrhages (if posterior limit of haemorrhage not visible, this is suggestive of orbital floor fracture).
- Examine the cornea for abrasions and lacerations; perform a Seidel test with fluorescein (Ch. 32) if there is any suspicion of a leak (from corneal or conjunctival wounds). Only central corneal abrasions tend to reduce visual acuity significantly.
- Look at the anterior chamber (AC). Note carefully the presence of cells (white or red), the presence of fibrin and also the AC depth relative to the other side (a shallow AC may suggest globe rupture). The depth of a *hyphaema* should be measured on the slitlamp carefully.
- Examine the iris, looking for evidence of traumatic *mydriasis* (differentiate carefully from a 3rd nerve palsy—check eye movements), sphincter rupture and *iridodialysis*.
- Check the intraocular pressure. A lower pressure than the contralateral eye is consistent with a traumatic iritis, but also with rupture of the globe. A hyphaema may result in elevated pressure.
- If not already done, ensure that an RAPD has been elicited before dilating the pupils.
- Examine the lens—traumatic cataracts can form very quickly. In addition, look for evidence of zonular damage in the form of *iridodonesis* and *phacodonesis*, by asking the patient to look to the side and then straight-ahead. If there is zonular instability, the lens and/or iris will wobble.
- Examine the vitreous for blood, *tobacco dust* and the presence or absence of a posterior vitreous detachment.
- Finally examine the retina. Look for areas of *commotio retinae* (much more obvious in a pigmented fundus), which are more commonly found inferiorly due to Bell's phenomenon, macular damage (e.g. traumatic macular hole), peripheral retinal tears, retinal dialyses and/or detachments, choroidal rupture and intraocular foreign bodies.
- A radiograph of the orbits is useful if there is a suspicion of an orbital floor fracture. In addition, posterior–anterior and lateral views are essential if an intraorbital foreign body is suspected. In the setting of busy eye casualty sessions, the author often sends patients for their radiographs after instilling mydriatic drops (provided that they are accompanied), examining the retina on their return.

Section 4
Ophthalmic investigations

Hess test

MJ Hawker

Introduction

The Hess chart is used to further investigate *incomitant* strabismus (where the squint angle changes depending on the direction of gaze). The test should be preceded by thorough clinical ophthalmic/oculomotor examination aimed at determining the cause of the strabismus.

There are two major types of defect causing incomitant strabismus:

- neurogenic/myogenic, e.g. 3rd, 4th, or 6th palsy, myasthenia gravis
- mechanical, e.g. dysthyroid eye disease, blow-out fracture.

It is possible to determine which type of defect is present from the Hess chart because they produce different patterns of deviation on the chart.

Theory and assumptions of the test

The test is performed with both eyes open, and with each eye fixing in turn. The test *dissociates* the eyes by providing a different coloured stimulus to each eye. Therefore, it provides no stimulus for fusion. The fixing eye is directed in different positions of gaze and the consequent position of gaze of the non-fixing eye is recorded. Therefore, the test plots out the effects of:

- Hering's law—during any *conjugate* eye movement (same direction), equal and simultaneous innervation flows to corresponding muscles (yoke muscles, e.g. left medial rectus, right lateral rectus) to contract.
- Sherrington's law—during contraction of an agonist (e.g. left lateral rectus), equal and simultaneous signal to relax is sent to the antagonist (e.g. left medial rectus).
- Primary deviation—the squint angle when fixing with the unaffected eye (e.g. the angle of right esotropia in right lateral rectus palsy when fixating with the left eye).
- Secondary deviation—the squint angle when fixing the affected eye (e.g. angle of left esotropia in right lateral rectus palsy when fixating with the right eye).

The test assumes that the fovea is used to fixate, that there is normal retinal correspondence, no suppression and that visual acuity is good enough to see the coloured lights used.

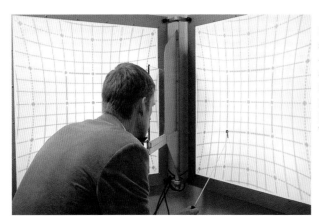

Fig. 36.1 The Lees screen. A mirror angled at 45° dissociates the eyes, allowing the plotting of the movements of one of the patient's eyes while the patient observes a target with the other eye.

Performing the test

The Hess screen is a grey board marked with a grid on which small red lights are individually illuminated. The patient wears red and green goggles, with the red goggle (which transmits red light and absorbs other wavelengths; = 'green filter') before the fixing eye. Only the fixing eye will therefore see the red light on the grid. The patient directs a green torchlight to where the non-fixing eye perceives the red light to be. Each screen consists of a central dot, an inner square of eight dots and an outer square of 16 dots (15° and 30° from the primary position, respectively). A similar test is performed using a Lees screen (two screens at 90° to each other, bisected by a mirror at 45° to achieve dissociation; Fig. 36.1). The results are plotted on a chart.

Interpreting the test

When looking at the chart, the deviation of the right eye (whilst fixing with left eye) is on the right side and vice versa. Each square on the chart equals 5° of arc. The chart is marked with the direction of action of each muscle to aid interpretation.

- Smaller chart indicates the eye with the underacting muscle (primary deviation).
- Larger chart indicates the eye with the overacting muscle (secondary deviation).
- Smaller chart shows greatest restriction in main direction of action of underacting muscle.
- Larger chart shows greatest expansion in main direction of action of yoke muscle (Hering's Law).
- Compare the position of each eye when the other eye is fixing in the primary position. Is there vertical deviation, e.g. right higher than left (right hypertropia) in a right 4th nerve palsy?

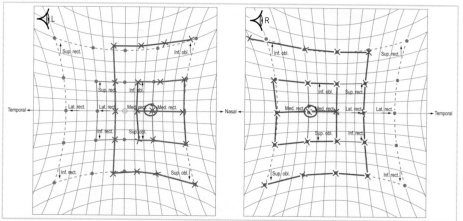

Fig. 36.2 A Hess test plot of a left lateral rectus palsy. The left eye's chart is smaller, indicating the laterality of the problem. The greatest restriction in movement is laterally, highlighting the paretic lateral rectus. The right chart is greatly expanded medially, this being the direction of action of the right medial rectus (the yoke muscle to the paretic left lateral rectus).

An example of a left lateral rectus palsy is shown in Figure 36.2.

Differences between neurogenic and mechanical causes

Mechanical causes tend to show:

- Deviation in primary position is not proportional to extent of limitation (e.g. in an orbital floor blow-out fracture causing tethering of the inferior rectus, the eye may be straight in the primary position and not show deviation until it elevates).
- Site of limited movement often opposite to where the cause is (tethering).
- Straight line of limitation when plotted on chart (neurogenic causes produce charts with curved lines indicating the boundary of limitation).

Evolution over time

As time passes, incomitant defects, particularly of neurogenic cause, become more *concomitant* (the angle of deviation differs less with changing positions of gaze). Following palsy of an agonist, there is concurrent overaction of the contralateral synergist (yoke) muscle (Hering's law). As a result of its unopposed action, the ipsilateral antagonist overacts, and with time undergoes contracture because of the deviation of the eye, which allows it to passively shorten. Contracture shows on the chart as an overaction. Since the direct antagonist of the affected muscle is acting unopposed this muscle requires less innervation. According to Hering's law, this results in less innervation to its yoke muscle, so a secondary underaction of the contralateral antagonist is seen. This combination of overactions and underactions serves to make the deviation between the eyes more concomitant.

For example, following a right 4th palsy the following occur:

- primary underaction of the ipsilateral agonist (right superior oblique)
- secondary overaction of the contralateral synergist/yoke muscle (left inferior rectus)
- overaction of the ipsilateral antagonist (right inferior oblique)
- secondary underaction of the contralateral antagonist (left superior rectus).

37

Fundus fluorescein angiography (FFA)

TLNH Kersey

Introduction

This investigation is an invasive test, which involves the intravenous injection of a fluorescent dye, to aid in the diagnosis of retinal conditions and planning of laser treatment. It is usually carried out by either a junior doctor or trained nurse practitioner in conjunction with a photographer.

Fluorescein is an orange water-soluble dye, whose molecules emit green light when stimulated by incident blue light. It is usually injected intravenously and as it passes through the retinal and choroidal circulations, a series of photographs are taken through the patient's dilated pupils. Occasionally, fluorescein is actually given orally, followed by a limited sequence of (later) photographs. It is often up to the junior doctor to gain consent from the patient and inject the dye, as well as to be available in the case of any adverse reaction.

For information regarding interpretation of fluorescein angiographic images, see Chapter 38 ('Fundus fluorescein angiography: an introduction to interpretation').

Indications

Fluorescein angiography is used most commonly in medical retina clinics to identify fundal lesions such as subretinal neovascular membranes, or to identify areas of microvascular leakage (e.g. as in proliferative diabetic retinopathy). Prior to requesting an FFA, it must be considered whether an angiogram will actually supply the extra information needed to clinch a diagnosis or change the management of a condition; many are requested unnecessarily. Anterior segment fluorescein angiography is occasionally used to investigate the anterior vasculature; the principles of fluorescence remain the same.

Principles and photographs

The procedure relies on the principle of fluorescence—the property that some molecules give off light energy of a longer wavelength when subjected to light of a shorter wavelength. Blue light of 490 nm is shone into the eye and fluorescein molecules emit green light of 530 nm, which is detected by the camera. This is achieved through a blue excitation filter for the camera flash and a green-yellow barrier filter in front of the (black and white) camera film or digital camera apparatus.

The photographer will initially take some red-free and colour fundus photographs of both eyes. After injection of the dye, a series of black and white photographs (of the requested eye only) will then be taken initially every few seconds for 25–30 seconds, then every minute or so in both eyes for about 5 minutes. Depending on the indication for the test, photographs are occasionally taken up to 30–40 minutes after injection of the dye.

Medical assessment

A medical history should be taken to exclude:

- cardiorespiratory pathology and severe hypertension
- previous adverse drug reactions
- previous anaphylaxis.

Consent

The patient is warned of the common side-effects of the dye:

- bright yellow discolouration of the skin and urine for several days, occasionally with photosensitivity
- a transient but strong nauseous reaction several seconds after the dye has been injected
- other effects including flushing, itching and excessive sneezing.

They should also be warned about more severe but rarer complications, including:

- bronchospasm
- anaphylaxis.

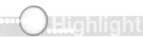

How to treat anaphylaxis

1. Remove the precipitating cause, i.e. stop injecting fluorescein.
2. Obtain urgent medical support (via nurses and switchboard).
3. Administer:
    - oxygen
    - 0.5 mg adrenaline (epinephrine) i.m. (i.e. 0.5 ml of 1:1000 solution)
    - colloid, e.g. Haemaccel 500 ml rapid infusion i.v.
    - antihistamine, e.g. 10 mg chlorphenamine i.v.
    - Hydrocortisone 200 mg i.v.
    - Consider nebulised salbutamol (5 mg) if severe bronchospasm.

Repeat adrenaline (epinephrine) every 10 min until improvement.

In view of the possibility of a severe reaction occurring, it is essential that you are familiar with the management of anaphylaxis and resuscitation techniques.

The procedure

The following description should allow an understanding of the steps involved:

- The pupils should be dilated adequately (usually with phenylephrine (2.5%) and tropicamide (1%)).
- Intravenous access should be gained with a cannula large enough to be of some use in the event of circulatory collapse (e.g. 21G). Venous access in the antecubital fossa allows a more rapid injection of fluorescein and is preferred in some departments, but is a little more uncomfortable for the patient.
- The dye should be drawn up to 5 ml of a 10% solution (this may vary locally, occasionally 2.5 ml used, sometimes 20% fluorescein). Gloves should be worn as the dye may stain skin for several days. (If you are unlucky enough to spill it on clothing, soaking in milk before washing will help.)
- At the photographer's beckoning, the dye is then injected rapidly with a saline flush to follow.
- As well as the standard resuscitation equipment, it is always worth having a sick bowl (e.g. kidney dish) to hand, in case the patient develops marked nausea and subsequent vomiting.

38

Fundus fluorescein angiography: an introduction to interpretation

SV Raman

Introduction

The property of fluorescence by the fluorescein molecule is utilised in this technique. Fluorescein emits light in the green region (wavelength 530 nm) of the spectrum when stimulated by light of wavelength at the blue end (490 nm) of the spectrum. Suitable filters (blue excitation filter, yellow-green barrier filter) are therefore incorporated in the camera to exploit this property in fluorescein angiography.

This chapter will provide a background to the understanding and interpretation of basic fluorescein angiographic images. For information concerning more general aspects of fluorescein angiography, including consent and safety issues, see Chapter 37.

Retinal physiology

In order to interpret a fundus angiogram, it is essential to understand some of the important anatomic and physiological aspects of the retina and choroid.

Retina

- The neurosensory retina can be divided into two layers: a vascular inner two-thirds and an avascular outer third.

- The outer plexiform layer forms the watershed zone between the vascular and avascular retina. The avascular outer retina receives its nourishment from the choroidal circulation.

- Normal retinal blood vessels do not leak fluorescein. This is due to the presence of a non-fenestrated capillary endothelium, which forms the *inner blood–retina barrier*.

- On fluorescein angiographic images, the macula is darker than the rest of the fundus due to tall and abundant melanin-containing retinal pigment epithelial (RPE) cells. It is also due to the absence of blood vessels in the region of the foveal avascular zone (FAZ), which measures approximately 350–500 μm in diameter.

- Tight junctional complexes (zonula occludens and zonula adherens) bind the RPE cells to one another. This forms the *outer blood–retina barrier*. Passage of fluorescein beyond this barrier suggests pathology.

Choroid

- The larger choroidal vessels do not leak fluorescein due to non-fenestrated endothelium.
- The choroidal capillaries leak fluorescein, but this cannot pass beyond a healthy RPE cell layer due to the presence of the outer blood–retinal barrier (see above).
- The dark RPE cells act as a natural optical barrier and make it difficult to interpret diseases of the choroid on the basis of fluorescein angiography (see 'ICG' box below).

Technical aspects of fluorescein angiography

- Fluorescein angiograms were traditionally captured, processed and read on 35 mm black and white film.
- With the advent of the digital era, more and more units are using a digital system. The angiogram results are read directly from the computer monitor or printed on a glossy photographic A4 sheet of paper.
- While looking at an angiogram result, it is important to look at the time sequence of the angiogram; this is usually printed in the right-hand corner or at the bottom of the frame. The elapsed time (since injection of the dye) is expressed in minutes and seconds.
- Fluorescein angiography is a dynamic study, involving two vascular networks: the short posterior ciliary vessels supplying the choroid (and indirectly the outer third of the retina) and the central retinal vessels supplying the inner two-thirds of the retina. A single angiogram frame by itself is not useful; complete frame-by-frame analysis (sometimes for up to 30–40 minutes) is necessary to understand and interpret the pathology.
- Stereoscopic images are occasionally requested. These are captured by taking two photographs of the same retinal area from slightly different positions, which are then fused together by the observer, providing a degree of stereopsis.

The normal angiogram

The normal angiogram (Fig. 38.1) can be broadly divided into five phases:

1. Choroidal
2. Arterial
3. Arteriovenous
4. Venous
5. The late phase.

- Fluorescein makes its appearance first in the choroidal circulation, usually 10–12 seconds after injection in a healthy young adult. This may take 12–15

Ophthalmic investigations

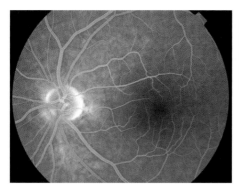

Fig. 38.1 A normal angiogram showing fluorescence of the retinal vessels and diffuse choroidal fluorescence. Note the normal relatively hypofluorescent macula (compare with the macula in Fig. 38.3).

seconds in an older individual, but the exact timing is dependent on other factors such as poor ventricular function, generalised atherosclerosis, etc. An inordinate delay may be seen with carotid artery stenosis (as seen in the ocular ischaemic syndrome).

- The central retinal artery begins to fill 1–3 seconds after the choroidal phase.

- Once the arteries have filled, the capillaries and veins begin to fill. This arteriovenous phase is characterised by a typical angiographic pattern known as *laminar flow*. The veins are fluorescent near their walls and darker in the centre. Within the next 5–10 seconds, the veins fill completely.

- The fluorescein starts to leave the retinal circulation at approximately 30 seconds after injection. Subsequent recirculation of fluorescein into the eye becomes weaker and less intense, as it gradually becomes redistributed around the body (making skin yellow, etc.) and subsequently eliminated (renal excretion) from the body. Nevertheless, the late phase of the angiogram gives valuable information, particularly in confirming cystoid macular oedema, and diagnosing occult subretinal neovascular membranes.

The abnormal angiogram

The abnormality in an angiogram is either a *hypofluorescent* or a *hyperfluorescent* area.

Hypofluorescence

- Hypofluorescence (Figs 38.2 and 38.3) can be due to either a reduction or an absence of the normal fluorescein filling of vessels (choroidal or retinal).

- The centre of the macula is normally hypofluorescent, due to the absence of retinal vessels, with the underlying choroidal fluorescence being blocked by the melanin and xanthophyll pigment of the retina.

- Absence of vascular tissue (e.g. an area of ischaemia due to a vein occlusion), or obstruction of a particular vessel with non-perfusion (e.g. in a branch arterial occlusion), will cause hypofluorescence.

- Pigment, blood, exudate and non-vascular tumours can block normal underlying fluorescence (of either the choroidal or retinal circulation, depending on

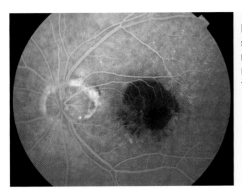

Fig. 38.2 Fluorescein angiogram showing hypofluorescence due to deep retinal blood. Note the normal overlying retinal vascular fluorescence, signifying that the blood is below the fluorescent vessels.

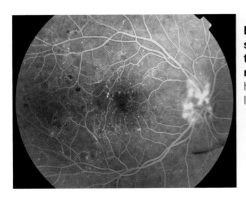

Fig. 38.3 Fluorescein angiogram showing a hypofluorescent macula due to macular ischaemia in diabetic retinopathy. In contrast, note the hyperfluorescent optic disc, which is due to leakage of fluorescein from new vessels.

the depth of the lesion). For example, subhyaloid blood (between retinal surface and vitreous body) will block both the retinal and choroidal fluorescence, whereas deep intra- or subretinal blood will cause hypofluorescence of the underlying choroidal circulation.

- The nature of blockage (blood, pigment, tumour or exudate) and the depth of the lesion can be inferred by clinical examination. A colour photograph usually accompanies an angiogram and careful examination of the combination of the two will help elucidate the nature of the lesion.

Hyperfluorescence

Hyperfluorescence can be due to leakage, staining, pooling and window defects.

- Hyperfluorescence due to leakage occurs with the presence of fluorescein dye in the extravascular compartment. Leakage, by definition, implies a defective blood–retina barrier (e.g. as seen in new vessels in proliferative diabetic retinopathy).

- In trying to spot leakage, it is necessary to follow the angiogram frame in a sequential manner and look for an increase in both the intensity and area of fluorescence (Fig. 38.4).

- In leakage, the increase in area of fluorescence is usually accompanied by the margin becoming slightly indistinct and fuzzy.

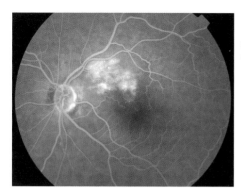

Fig. 38.4 Late frame of an angiogram showing leakage in a branch retinal vein occlusion. Note the fuzzy margin.

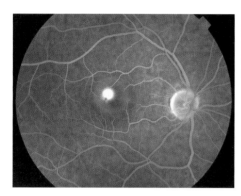

Fig. 38.5 Late frame of an angiogram showing pooling of fluorescein in the subretinal space (a case of central serous chorioretinopathy).

- Pooling of fluorescein occurs either in the subretinal or sub-RPE space (central serous retinopathy, wet age-related macular degeneration) (Fig. 38.5).

- Some structures tend to retain fluorescein, so producing staining, e.g. scar tissue (such as a disciform scar) and drusen.

- A localised (as in atrophic macular degeneration) or generalised (as in high myopia) lack of RPE unmasks the underlying choroidal fluorescence, producing an RPE window defect; in other words, you can see through the window in the RPE to the choroid. The difference in hyperfluorescence seen in leakage and window defects can often be appreciated by carefully studying the accompanying colour photographs; areas of atrophic macular degeneration are usually easy to spot.

Further Information

ICG angiography

ICG (indocyanine green) angiography is an investigation used in some centres to provide more information about the choroidal circulation (and pathology resulting from the choroid, e.g. subretinal neovascular membranes). ICG also fluoresces but does so in the infrared range of wavelengths, and in response to a different stimulating light source to fluorescein. Normal RPE pigments do not block the infrared radiation; thus, by using a specially adapted camera to capture the emitted infrared rays, information can be gleaned about the choroidal circulation, which would otherwise be invisible to fluorescein angiography. This technique takes longer to perform than FFA, but has provided much useful information about many conditions originally thought to be retinal in origin (e.g. central serous chorioretinopathy (CSCR)).

39

Corneal topography

JP Kersey

Background

Corneal topography was originally assessed using a Placido disc. This handheld device had a series of concentric black and white rings on a large disc, with a central viewing hole. With bright illumination, this produced a series of corneal reflexes, which could be examined through the viewing hole and any astigmatism visualised. Though still available in many departments, it is not commonly used today.

Cameras were later mounted behind the disc to photograph the reflexes, so allowing a record to be kept for comparison with further and subsequent examinations. This was not very objective and more recently computers have been used to analyse the patterns created by these corneal reflexes to produce quantitative mapping of the corneal curvature (computer-assisted videokeratoscopy). More recently, in order to aid interpretation, a colour scheme has been superimposed, with red implying a steeper, and blue a flatter, curvature.

Application

Corneal topography has arisen from the need to improve on the results of standard keratometry (Ch. 16), which only produces useful results for patients with regular astigmatism; patients with irregular astigmatism are not adequately assessed with this technique. Modern corneal topographers measure over 5000 points across the whole cornea and 1000 within the central 3 mm, so providing a large amount of information regarding corneal curvature in both irregular and regular astigmatism.

Indications for topography include keratoconus (shown below), corneal scarring and the planning of cataract surgery in patients with irregular (or high regular) astigmatism. Corneal scarring can be due to many causes, such as trauma, previous infections, corneal dystrophies or surgery (such as penetrating keratoplasty). Following corneal graft surgery, topography can identify any tight sutures, allowing the removal of individual sutures to reduce post-operative astigmatism.

Techniques

The machine is usually mounted in front of a standard chin rest. The patient places head on the rest and looks into the machine. The reflexes are then focused (the method of focusing varies with the machine) and a reading taken. A printout of the results is then obtained.

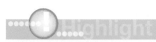

Tips and pitfalls

- The patient must be looking straight ahead.
- The corneal reflexes must be centralised to allow interpretation.
- The patient must have a wide palpable aperture and not blink during the reading.
- Get the patient to blink several times prior to taking the readings and be specific about telling the patient to look straight ahead with a big wide stare.
- Occasionally it may be necessary to use artificial teardrops to achieve an adequate reflectance.

Interpretation

The different colours in the images produced represent the corneal steepness at various measured points across the cornea. Different indices can be used to alter the calculations made by the machine to produce the colour map. The basic variables are described below. Common examples are shown at the end of this chapter.

Relative and absolute scales

In an absolute scale, the colours are the same for certain curvatures or powers, with the steps between the colours also being fixed. This, however, is only true for one type of machine and the scales do vary between machines. Thus, it is vital to check the scale prior to trying to interpret the map. In a relative scale, however, the colour range is adjusted so that the whole colour range covers the curvature or power range of the particular eye being examined. This means that while more information is available on small changes in that cornea, the scales may be different even on the same machine measuring the same eye on different occasions.

Power and radius scales

The refractive strength of the cornea at various points can be measured using either the corneal radius of curvature or the corneal power. These scales are inversely proportional to each other, with a smaller radius of curvature indicating a higher corneal power at that point. Both of these scales are derived from the first differentials of the corneal height at that point. The radius of curvature is more accurate than the power measurement, but the latter is generally used more in clinical practice.

Axial versus tangential maps

Axial maps use colour to identify the dioptric power of the cornea at specific points on the corneal surface. Such a map is usually easier to interpret, but makes several assumptions about the spherical nature of the cornea. This has

Ophthalmic investigations

the effect of smoothing out some of the minor changes in corneal curvature. Tangential maps use colour to denote change in corneal curvature and as such are better able to demonstrate minor changes. The calculations used to produce a tangential map make less assumptions about the shape of the cornea, allowing it to be more accurate in measuring the peripheral corneal shape.

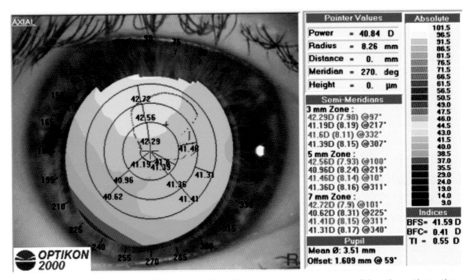

Fig. 39.1 Normal corneal topography. Although there is some mild astigmatism, the dioptric values marked are very similar and are of no clinical significance. (Image courtesy of Optikon 2000 SpA.)

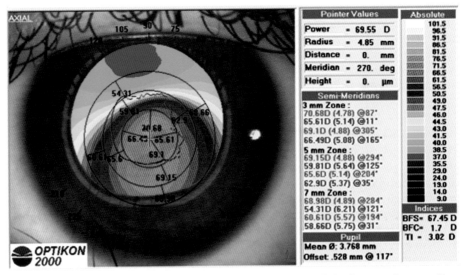

Fig. 39.2 Topography of keratoconus. Note the large inferiorly decentred cone with very high dioptric values marked in a bright red (steep) colour. (Image courtesy of Optikon 2000 SpA.)

Other machines

There are many different types of machine available and many use different software; familiarisation with your local machine and its printouts is therefore essential.

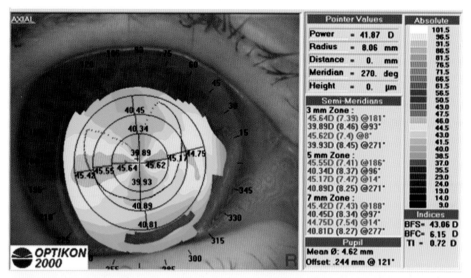

Fig. 39.3 Topography of marked regular (against-the-rule) astigmatism. The difference in corneal power in the vertical and horizontal meridia appears to be in the order of 5.5 D. (Image courtesy of Optikon 2000 SpA.)

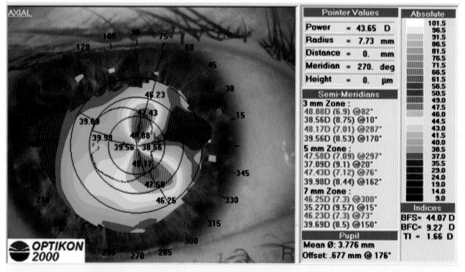

Fig. 39.4 Topography of irregular astigmatism in a patient after penetrating keratoplasty. Note that the axes of the (≈10 D) of astigmatism present are not perpendicular; satisfactory spectacle correction would probably be impossible. (Image courtesy of Optikon 2000 SpA.)

Images

As different patterns are characteristic of different diseases, several of the more common conditions are shown in Figures 39.1–39.4. The central cornea is typically steeper than the periphery in normal corneas. In the images shown, the steeper areas of the cornea are in yellow/red while the flatter areas are green/blue; a key to the colour schemes of other machines is usually to be found on the various individual printouts.

40

Electrodiagnostics

JP Kersey

Introduction

Electrodiagnostic testing can help considerably in the diagnosis of several specific ocular conditions. This chapter will give an overview of the various tests available and some idea of basic interpretation. Further reading at the end will guide those who would like to know more.

Electro-oculogram (EOG)

The electro-oculogram test (Fig. 40.1) is one of the few electrodiagnostic tests which, in conjunction with the appropriate clinical picture, can be used diagnostically.

- Electrodes are placed over the medial and lateral canthi of the eye to be measured.
- The patient is asked to look from side to side at a steady rate.
- The cornea is positive in charge relative to the retina and as the eye moves the charge in the electrodes fluctuates.
- This fluctuating electrical signal is amplified and recorded.
- Measurements are taken in both the light- and dark-adapted states.

There is a large amount of variation between individuals regarding absolute readings. The light response is divided by the dark response and the result is expressed as a percentage (Arden ratio), so allowing comparison between individuals and between recordings for the same individual.

Further Information

Arden ratio

Arden ratio = light peak /dark trough × 100 (normal ≥ 185%).

Further Information

Common clinical responses

- Absent EOG, but present ERG (see below): Best's disease.
- Absent light rise: retinitis pigmentosa.

Ophthalmic investigations

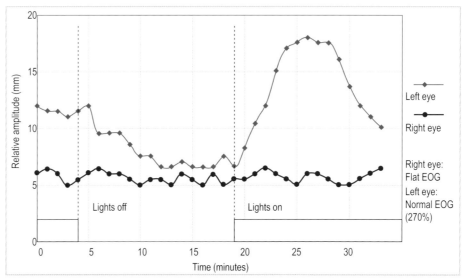

Fig. 40.1 An electro-oculogram showing a normal light rise in the left eye with an absent light rise in the right.

Electroretinogram (ERG)

The electroretinogram (Fig. 40.2) is a measurement of the retinal electrical response to a light stimulus. It is affected by the adaptive state of the eye and the type of stimulus presented. It is therefore possible to produce a cone ERG (30 Hz flicker in bright conditions, photopic) or a rod ERG (dim flash in the dark adapted eye, scotopic).

- The basic ERG is performed using an electrode placed in contact with the cornea and a second reference electrode placed on the forehead. The corneal contact electrode can be in the form either of a contact lens with an embedded electrode, or a gold foil.
- The stimulus is then administered while recording occurs.

The response contains two main waves: the negative *a* wave and the positive *b* wave. The *a* wave predominantly arises from the photoreceptors while the *b* wave arises predominantly from the inner retina, mainly the Müller cells.

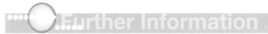

Common clinical results

- Negative ERG: preserved *a* wave, but reduced *b* wave is found in many conditions which include: central retinal artery occlusion and congenital stationary night blindness.
- No ERG response: Batten's disease, Leber's amaurosis.
- Increased *a* wave: albinism.

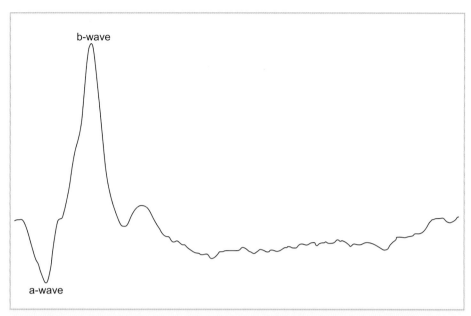

b-wave

a-wave

Fig. 40.2 An example of a normal photopic electroretinogram in response to a bright white flash, showing a negative *a* wave followed by a positive *b* wave.

Pattern electroretinogram (PERG)

Pattern electroretinogram (Fig. 40.3) is the retinal electrical response to a patterned stimulus (usually a reversing chequerboard) and is predominantly a measure of central retinal and ganglion cell function.

The corneal electrode needs to avoid the visual axis, so a gold foil is commonly used and the reference electrode must be placed on the ipsilateral temple or outer canthus, to avoid contamination from the cortical-evoked potential, which can occur if the electrode is on the forehead or ear.

The PERG shows three responses: an initial negative wave N 35, a positive wave P 50 (macular photoreceptors) and finally a second negative wave N 95 (ganglion cell layer). Features of the PERG used clinically include: the size of the P 50 component, the amplitude of N 95, the N 95:P 50 ratio and the P 50 latency.

Further Information

Common clinical responses

- Abnormal PERG, normal ERG: abnormal macular function (e.g. Stargardt macular dystrophy).
- Abnormal PERG, abnormal ERG: generalised rod/cone dystrophy.

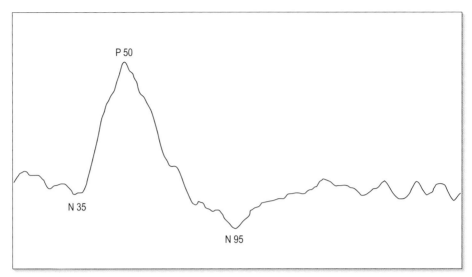

Fig. 40.3 An example of a pattern electroretinogram, showing an initial positive P 50 response, followed by the negative N 95 wave.

Multifocal electroretinogram (mfERG)

Standard ERG techniques and their varying protocols allow differentiation between pathology of rod or cone photoreceptors (as in scotopic and photopic responses), but are unable to facilitate spatial localisation of pathology. However, in MFERG (Fig. 40.4), a computer is used to mathematically isolate specific spatial areas of the retina according to specific temporal patterns of stimulation. To allow this, the stimulus screen is typically divided into 103 (sometimes 61) hexagonal elements, each element being accorded a particular size in order to stimulate approximately the same number of receptors. Each element flashes in a pseudo-random sequence, giving the appearance of a flickering screen; however, by correlating the stimulus sequence with the ERG signal, an individual ERG signal for each of the elements can be obtained (providing that central fixation is maintained).

The data may be displayed in various ways, either numerically or as a waveform, or the amplitude values may be shown as a three-dimensional colour figure (as in Fig. 40.4).

Visual-evoked potential (VEP)

VEP (Fig. 40.5) is a measurement of cortical electrical response to either a flash or pattern stimulus. It is predominantly a measure of optic nerve function and can be used to quantify approximate visual acuity. It requires electrodes to be placed over both the occipital areas.

The normal pattern VEP response includes a negative response N 75, a positive response P 100 and a second negative response N 135. The P 100 latency is also measured.

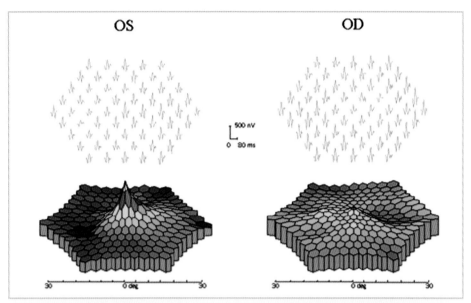

Fig. 40.4 An example of multifocal electroretinography. Compared to the normal left eye, the right eye shows abnormal macular responses, with focal reductions in the central waveforms and a corresponding change in the three-dimensional colour figure.

As the stimulus is presented monocularly and responses over both occipital cortices are measured, this allows an indication of the degree of crossover at the chiasm. Use of half-field stimuli, taking advantage of the anatomy of visual processing, can further isolate pathology. Furthermore, *multifocal* VEPs hold great promise for the future of electrodiagnostics.

Further Information

Common clinical responses

- Delayed VEP: demyelination.
- Enhanced cross-over: albinism.
- Normal VEP can help identify hysterics and malingerers.

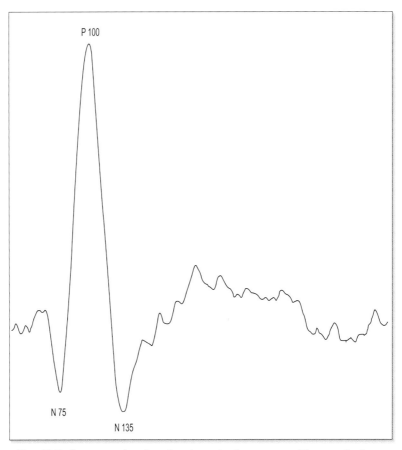

Fig. 40.5 An example of a visual-evoked response. The graph shows an initial N 75 negative response, followed by the positive P 100 and the ensuing negative N 135 wave.

41

Testing for stereopsis

MJ Hawker

Stereoscopic vision

Stereopsis is the ability to fuse slightly dissimilar images (viewed from different angles by the two eyes) to create the perception of depth. Stereopsis is the pinnacle of Worth's three grades of binocular vision (simultaneous perception, fusion, stereopsis). Firstly, it requires simultaneous perception from both eyes which is often absent if there is suppression or amblyopia. Secondly, it requires the ability to fuse images from the two eyes. Sensory fusion allows the patient to superimpose the images from each eye into a composite image. Motor fusion is the ability to move the eyes through a range of vergence movements to achieve sensory fusion. Normal simultaneous perception and sensory and motor fusion achieves binocular single vision (BSV). BSV therefore occurs when the image falls on corresponding retinal elements in the two eyes. Stereopsis, which cannot occur without BSV, requires the images to fall on slightly disparate retinal elements of the two eyes, but within Panum's fusional area, otherwise diplopia results.

Stereoacuity is graded according to the minimum angle of image disparity, which gives the appreciation of depth. Normal stereoacuity is approximately 60 seconds of arc or better; however, an individual with very good stereoacuity may achieve 15 seconds of arc or better. Maximum stereoacuity is found at the macula, where the resolving power of the eye is at its best.

Clinical tests of stereoacuity

Depth perception may be achieved in two ways:

- Stereopsis.
- Monocular depth cues (used in the absence of BSV), including:
  - light and shade
  - perspective and the relative size of objects
  - parallax.

A good test of stereoacuity will therefore avoid giving monocular clues.

Lang two-pencil test

This is a test for gross stereopsis. The patient attempts to place a vertical pencil on top of one held by the examiner. Patients with stereopsis will find this task much easier than those without.

Ophthalmic investigations

Frisby stereotest

This consists of clear Perspex plates of different thicknesses (6 mm, 3 mm, 1 mm; see Fig. 41.1). On each plate there are four squares filled with random shapes printed on the front surface. In one of the squares a 'hidden' circle of shapes is printed on the back surface of the Perspex. This creates disparity. Each test plate should be held at 40 cm and tests for stereopsis of 340, 170 and 55 seconds of arc according to the three thicknesses. The test is useful for young children, but care must be taken to present the plate perpendicularly, otherwise monocular clues (e.g. parallax) are given.

Random dot stereograms

Random dot stereograms comprise images which are formed by the displacement of random dots in relation to each other. Each eye views a different collection of random dots, an image only being perceived when both eyes view the dots simultaneously. The grade of stereopsis is measured by altering the degree of displacement between the random dots. Random dot stereogram tests include:

- Lang stereotest
- TNO stereotest.

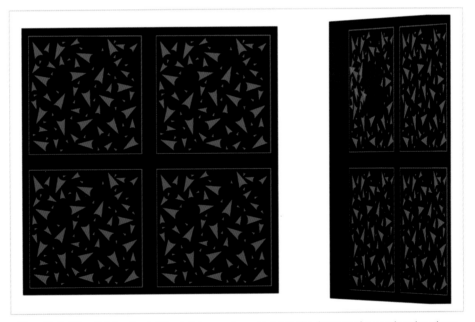

Fig. 41.1 The Frisby test. The left image is seen from the front and no uniocular clues are given as to which square has the elevated images. On the right, the test has been turned so that it is viewed obliquely from the side. To illustrate the elevated images better, they are displayed in red in this example.

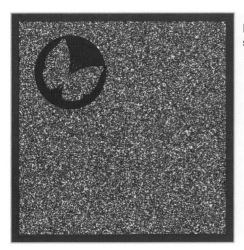

Fig 41.2 An example of one of the shapes seen in the TNO test.

Lang stereotest

A cylindrical grating is used to present random dot stereograms to the right and left eyes. The two images are fused and the disparity evokes stereopsis. The test is viewed at 40 cm and must be held perpendicularly to prevent monocular clues. A star, which can be seen without stereopsis, is used as a control image and a car, elephant and moon test stereopsis from 1200 to 550 seconds of arc (at the prescribed distance).

TNO stereotest

Computer-generated random dots are printed as red and green anaglyphs (Fig. 41.2). The patient wears red and green glasses so that each eye views separate anaglyphs. The test consists of three gross stereotests, a suppression plate and three graded plates testing stereopsis from 480 to 15 seconds of arc. It is the most accurate test of stereopsis as it provides no monocular clues.

Linear polarisation stereotests

Polaroid filter glasses are worn to enable each eye to view separate, disparate images (vectographs). The targets consist of two superimposed views, one emitting a vertical image of polarised light, the other a horizontal one. Each image is viewed by separate eyes. Slight disparity between the images evokes stereopsis. A well-known example is the Titmus test.

Titmus test

This consists of two plates. The 'Wirt fly' tests for gross stereopsis, which is confirmed if the wings of the fly are perceived as standing out from the body. The second plate consists of nine boxes, each containing four circles, and three rows of animals. One circle in each box appears to stand out, and grades stereoacuity up to 40 seconds of arc. The image of one animal in each row also stands out, and grades stereoacuity up to 100 seconds of arc.

Ophthalmic investigations

Synoptophore

Stereopsis can also be assessed on the synoptophore with:

- Graded stereoscopic slides containing two disparate images. These test gross stereopsis.
- Braddick slides are forms of random dot stereograms, each slide stimulating slightly disparate retinal points of each eye, resulting in depth perception.

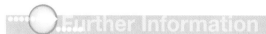

Further Information

Warning: The use of a dissociative stereoscopic test can break down a patient with a phoria to a manifest squint (tropia). In these patients, a non-dissociative test would be more appropriate (e.g. Frisby test).

Section 5
Common ophthalmic surgical procedures

42

An introduction to cataract surgery

JP Kersey

Introduction and a brief history

Cataract surgery has changed dramatically over the last 15 years. The three major types of operation performed are discussed below. While some senior ophthalmologists may remember the days of intracapsular cataract surgery (ICCE), this is now only performed routinely in a few areas of the developing world.

ICCE

This procedure involved extracting the lens in its entirety, capsular bag and all. It involved a large corneal incision, a recovery time of weeks to months and was not compatible with a posterior chamber intraocular lens. The patients were therefore left aphakic, requiring contact lenses or very high *plus* lens spectacles (+10 to +12 D).

The next advance in cataract surgery was to try and remove the lens, but leave behind the capsular bag, so allowing the insertion of a posterior chamber intraocular lens. This was called an extracapsular cataract extraction (ECCE).

ECCE

This procedure involved an incision of about one-third of the corneal circumference; however, the reduction in vitreous loss rates meant a considerable improvement in recovery time. This led to day-case cataract extraction becoming a more viable prospect. A jagged hole was made in the anterior capsule and the lens nucleus expressed through the incision in the cornea. This was usually performed via a rocking action and the delivery in unskilled hands was difficult to control. The visual outcomes were much better than seen in ICCE, but the drive for smaller incision procedures led to the adoption of phacoemulsification as the gold standard operation. With the advent of newer phacoemulsification machines on the market, visual outcomes have continued to improve.

Phacoemulsification (Phaco)

This procedure allows the nucleus to be broken up and aspirated through incisions of 4 mm or less. These wounds are self-sealing and so do not require sutures. They also have a lower astigmatic effect and so both recovery and visual outcomes have improved. Initially, however, increased damage to the corneal endothelium was occurring but this has been reduced with the use of better viscoelastic substances and an improvement in machine technology, so allowing a reduction in phaco power and the time needed to remove a standard nucleus.

Although success rates for cataract surgery are now very impressive, phaco techniques are still evolving; some centres have taken to using bimanual techniques, allowing microincision (2 mm or less) surgery, with potential improvements in postoperative astigmatism. Unfortunately, at the current time, intraocular lens technology is such that most microincisions still need to be enlarged after phacoemulsification to allow placement of a lens, limiting the utility of such a technique.

43

Cataract surgery preassessment

JP Kersey

Introduction

Increasingly, preoperative assessment is being performed in nurse- or optometrist-led clinics. However, it is certainly important to understand the principles involved as they will influence the choice of lens power used for the operation. In addition, preassessment of such patients forms an integral part of the Royal College part II Examination.

The assessment

There are four main parts to preoperative assessment of cataract patients:

1. General ophthalmic and medical assessment

This is usually performed in clinic and involves taking a thorough history to identify whether the patient has any visual symptoms, which would be improved by cataract surgery. Most surgery is carried out under local or topical anaesthesia; however, if the patient will need a general anaesthetic, suitability for that will also have to be established (see Ch. 47, 'Anaesthesia for ocular surgery').

General anaesthesia is often more suitable for patients with extreme anxiety, orthopnoea (provided the anaesthetist is willing), marked tremor, mental health problems, high myopes (due to risk of perforation of the globe during peribulbar anaesthesia) or in the occasional case of bilateral cataract surgery. General anaesthesia cases are often considered more appropriate opportunities for training of junior staff.

It is also important to establish whether the patient is anticoagulated. If so, then surgery (and local anaesthesia) will usually be safe if recent INRs are consistently in the range of 2–3. If not, an INR on the day of surgery should be checked; check your local unit policy.

2. Examination of the eye

The eye must be examined in the dilated state, as this will give an indication of the ease of the operation, as well as affording a clearer view of the posterior pole. Ideally, the intraocular pressures should be documented prior to dilatation. In addition, pay attention to factors such as marked blepharitis, which must be treated prior to the day of surgery. Some units use preoperative topical antibiotic eyedrops for every patient—ensure that you are aware of local protocol.

Factors that will make the operation more difficult (see Ch. 46, 'Spotting the difficult cataract') or potentially compromise the visual outcome (such as macular degeneration) should also be documented clearly. Until you are sure of the local criteria, it is important to consult with a senior colleague before listing a patient for surgery.

3. Measuring the eye (biometry)

It is an excellent idea to ask one of the nurses to show you how to use the biometry equipment, as you may be asked to use it if faced with a particularly difficult case! There are three main factors that need to be taken into account to calculate the power of intra-ocular lens needed for a particular eye. (For more detailed information on ocular biometry, see Ch. 7.)

(i) Patient's spectacle prescription and future requirements

The current spectacle prescription will be needed, as will information on whether the patient has a cataract in the other eye and wishes to have surgery on that eye as well. The final refractive outcome of the two eyes needs to be discussed. Most patients would like to be left emmetropic, thus hopefully not needing distance glasses. However, some patients, particularly myopes, would prefer to be left with spectacle-free reading vision, and a target refraction of −2.5 to −3 D would therefore be appropriate.

If the patient is left with a difference of more than 2–3 D between the two eyes, then spectacle correction may lead to an unacceptable level of *aniseikonia* (difference in retinal image size between the two eyes) and thus diplopia. The only reason for leaving a patient hypermetropic is if the other eye is significantly hypermetropic, and the patient only wants an operation on one eye.

(ii) *k* readings

k readings (Ch. 16) are a measure of corneal curvature and are usually described as K1 (the more horizontal) and K2 (the more vertical). Although initially measured using a manual keratometer (such as the Javal–Schiötz type), automated keratometers are now increasingly being used.

Example

Keratometry

Keratometry readings are recorded as dioptric power along an axis.
For example:

K1 43.50 D @ 175°

K2 44.00 D @ 85°

In this example, the difference between the two readings is 0.5 D, representing 0.5 D of corneal astigmatism.

Large differences indicate significant corneal astigmatism and should be checked against the patient's spectacle prescription, or unaided visual acuity. In an otherwise healthy eye (6/6 potential), 1 D of ametropia would reduce vision to around 6/18. 1 D of astigmatism will reduce it by half that (i.e. to around 6/9).

(iii) Axial length

This is still often measured using an A scan ultrasound machine, but is increasingly being automated using partial coherence laser interferometry (e.g. Zeiss IOL Master). The results are recorded as axial length in millimetres, with the mean of 5 or 10 measurements usually being used in the biometry calculations. Any significant differences between the two eyes (0.2–0.4 mm) should be checked against the patient's refraction; large differences may imply measuring errors.

4. Consent

Although not definitive, the following list contains the most important risks that may be discussed prior to surgery, including the commonest and most serious complications. Some patients, of course, do not want to listen to the long list of possible and dreadful complications; an often acceptable abbreviation is to warn them of the two major groups of risk, i.e. loss of vision and the need for another operation to try and correct complications.

- Postoperative need for glasses (especially reading glasses), dependent on planned postoperative refraction.
- Posterior capsule opacity (in one-third to half of patients).
- An expected poor visual outcome as a result of ocular comorbidity.
- Infection, rarely endophthalmitis (1:1000).
- Visual loss and 'blindness'.
- An increased risk of retinal detachment at any point after surgery.
- Cystoid macular oedema.
- Postoperative uveitis.
- Diplopia if there is a significant difference in refraction between the two eyes.
- Vitreous loss (leading to a second operation if dropped nucleus occurs).
- Corneal decompensation if Fuch's dystrophy is present.
- Suprachoroidal haemorrhage, especially in the case of planned ECCE surgery.
- The mentioning of visual loss in the other eye from sympathetic ophthalmia remains controversial but is standard practice in some countries (e.g. Australia).

Marking of eyes

It is standard practice prior to surgery in many hospitals to mark the forehead of the patient above the eye to be operated. This is increasingly likely to become routine practice in all hospitals as a clinical governance issue; check your local unit policy.

Phacoemulsification surgery

JP Kersey

Introduction

Phacoemulsification (phaco) involves the use of ultrasound to break up the cataractous nucleus to allow its extraction through a small incision.

A phaco hand-piece is currently a single instrument, which irrigates, aspirates and delivers an ultrasonic wave, which breaks up the lens. The vibrating phaco tip would heat up during constant use, which could potentially burn the cornea at the point where the tip passes through the corneal incision. This heating effect is therefore reduced by using a silicone rubber sleeve, utilising the irrigating fluid (balanced salt solution (BSS), different from normal saline) as a coolant running between the phaco tip and the sleeve, thus preventing much of the heat passing to the cornea. The lens remnants are aspirated up the centre of the tip and are removed from the eye.

Control of fluid flowing into and out of the eye is imperative for maintaining the anterior chamber (AC) depth. This is mainly dependent on the height of the irrigation bottle; the higher the bottle, the greater the intraocular pressure and the greater the AC depth. If the AC shallows, then the amount of room available for manipulation of the nuclear fragments is reduced, making the procedure considerably more difficult.

Stages of the procedure

It is now a College requirement in the UK to have completed a microsurgical skills course prior to starting intraocular surgery. For information contact the College (see 'Useful Contacts', p. 287).

There are eight main stages in a routine cataract procedure.

1. Preparing the eye

This varies considerably between hospitals and even between consultants within the same department. The fundamentals involve reducing the microbial load in the fornices and the use of a drape and speculum to remove the eyelashes from the surgical field.

- Povidone-iodine (5%) is almost universally used prior to surgery and is placed in the lower conjunctival fornix. It is the only method which has been proven to reduce endophthalmitis. Most surgeons also clean around the eye with the same solution or similar disinfectant. This does make the area damp and thorough drying of the eyelids will aid subsequent correct placement of the drape.

- Draping is definitely an art. There are several methods but the principle is to get the drape on with the eyelids as wide apart as possible, with the eyelashes

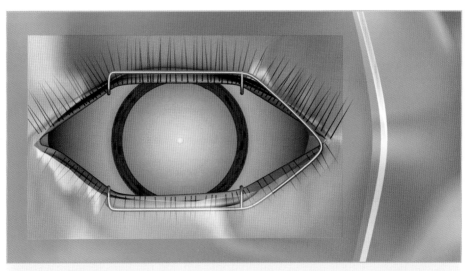

Fig. 44.1 Draping the eye. The lower surface of the drape is placed over the eye, with the patient keeping the eye open at all times. In this way the lashes are stuck down onto the lid skin and out of the operating field. The drape is then cut from the medial to the lateral canthus and a speculum inserted to keep the lids apart.

sticking to the drape and therefore away from the globe (Fig. 44.1). An incision is made through the drape closer to the lower lid than the upper one.

- The speculum is inserted so that the drape is reflected around the lid margins and often into the fornices. In the absence of akinesia, it is easiest to get the patient to look in the opposite direction to the lid that you are trying to place the speculum into, e.g. down if you are placing the upper part of the speculum. The upper lashes are the most important to cover completely with the drape, as you will be placing instruments in and out of the eye over this area the most.

2. Corneal incisions

There are several methods of corneal wound construction and it is a good idea to practise as many as possible to see which works best for you. The easiest way of doing this is to watch the consultant that you are working for and do it his or her way. As you rotate between consultants/surgeons, you will have to change techniques and will gain a broad experience of wound construction. The principles remain the same and there are balances to be struck between making the operation easier for you and getting the best visual result for the patient.

Most surgeons now use a single-use keratome which has a fixed width, designed to fit the phaco hand-piece being used. These vary in size from 2.5 to 3.5 mm, the commonest being close to 3 mm. Ask the theatre staff about the size of the instruments, as they will have important implications for the method of IOL insertion.

When making the wound, take care not to damage the underlying anterior capsule of the lens (although some surgeons *deliberately* use such a technique to initiate their capsulorhexis).

Common ophthalmic surgical procedures

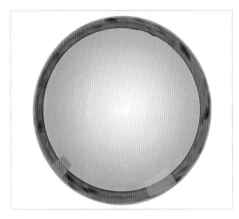

Fig. 44.2 Example of wound construction. Corneal incisions are deliberately made at an angle to the corneal surface in order to increase the length of the *tunnel* through the corneal stroma, producing a self-sealing wound and the characteristic square-shaped incision. In this diagram, the main incision is blue and the side-port is red.

Wound construction

- *Scleral tunnel.* This is a less common approach and involves forming a scleral pocket behind the limbus and tunnelling forward to the limbus. It is astigmatically neutral and the risk of wound leak is very low. It is a useful technique where subsequent contact lens placement (e.g. for macular laser treatment) is highly likely.

- *Corneal incisions:*

  - One-stage incision—a direct stab incision usually at the limbus, ideally 2–3 mm long.

  - Two-stage incision—an initial vertical incision into the limbus to create a lip and the second stage forming the tunnel in a similar method to a one-stage incision.

  - Three-stage incision—a vertical incision and a short tunnel within the stroma, almost parallel to the epithelium, which is followed by a more direct entrance into the eye.

Wound placement

For a discussion about the optical principles involved in the choice of incision site, see Chapter 4 ('Further concepts in astigmatism').

The example in Figure 44.2 shows the view that a right-handed surgeon would have through the operating microscope, with the blue incision representing the main wound and the red incision representing the side-port. The easiest position for the main wound is 10°–15° anticlockwise from the axis on which you are sitting. Other wounds occasionally need to be made and these are usually made after the insertion of viscoelastic. It is very difficult to make an incision into a soft eye.

3. Injection of viscoelastic

There are several different types of viscoelastic and they have differing properties:

- HPMC (hydroxy-propyl methyl cellulose) is the cheapest and is often made by a regional manufacturing pharmacy, such as at Moorfields Eye Hospital. It is much thicker than saline and as it has a higher surface tension, it will not leave the eye as readily as BSS. This means it will maintain the anterior chamber shape for longer, allowing procedures such as the capsulorhexis to be performed. It also has good optical properties and can be placed onto the cornea to reduce the need for regular watering (usually a task for junior ophthalmologists).

- Sodium hyaluronate. This is available in several types:
  - The standard formulation (e.g. Healon), providing good AC depth for the majority of cataract procedures. It is more viscous than HPMC and so will maintain the AC deeper for longer. However, it will need topping up during a prolonged procedure and a watch must be kept on the AC depth.
  - A high molecular weight variant (e.g. Healon GV), which is particularly useful for shallow ACs, as it allows more space and again has a higher surface tension. It stays in the AC more readily than the standard formulation, but is more difficult to remove at the end of the operation. Such variants are very useful for teaching inexperienced surgeons techniques such as the capsulorhexis, as they afford a much lower likelihood of the capsulorhexis extending peripherally.
  - 'Viscoadaptive' agents have been designed to be a compromise between the two above and their use is increasing, the expense being the main reason that they are not routinely used in most units.

4. Continuous curvilinear capsulorhexis (CCC)

This is probably one of the most difficult parts of the cataract operation to perfect. It requires the tearing of a near perfect circle in the anterior lens capsule. Initiation of the tear is usually performed by a sharp object, such as a needle, making a radial incision in the capsule around 2 mm in length. One edge of the tear is then lifted and folded over (Fig. 44.3) before extending the tear using one of two techniques:

- capsulorhexis forceps
- needle CCC.

Capsulorhexis forceps

With this technique, forceps are used to hold the edge of the capsular fold to allow it to be torn in a curvilinear manner. The direction of the tear is critical to maintain a consistent circular shape (Fig. 44.4). If the direction of the tear is too straight, the tear will move toward the periphery producing too large a capsulorhexis or, in extremis, a posterior capsule tear (not good). If the tear is too

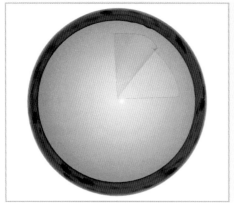

Fig. 44.3 Continuous curvilinear capsulorhexis (CCC): initial incision.
A capsulorhexis is created in the anterior capsule by using a sharp instrument to make an incision from the centre of the capsule towards the pupil margin. The capsule is then torn tangentially to create a flap.

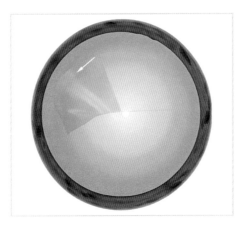

Fig. 44.4 Continuous curvilinear capsulorhexis (CCC): extension. The flap is extended to complete a circular capsulorhexis by repeatedly regrasping the flap at the tearing edge and tearing tangentially (see arrow). Best results are achieved when the entire flap is folded back and the folded edge remains perpendicular to the torn edge.

central, the capsulorhexis will be too small. (This technique is best practised in a non-threatening environment. This includes plastic eyes in a wet-lab or on tomatoes which have been placed into almost boiling water for a few minutes. The latter model is not ideal and has the risk of scalding (!), but is at least cheap and easily available.)

Needle CCC

This is the more difficult technique initially, but can have its advantages in skilled hands. There are various shapes and sizes of CCC needles (cystotomes) or you can bend your own (27 G) needle. It is worth putting the needle on the end of a syringe of viscoelastic so you can top up the AC easily if needed. The smaller size of the instrument means there is often a reduced rate of viscoelastic escape. The art is to catch the flap with just enough downward pressure to allow you to move it without disturbing the underlying lens material, which would otherwise obscure your view of the flap edge. It is a sideward stroking motion that works best.

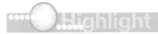

Highlight

CCC tips

The main difficulties are due to not maintaining a good AC depth. If the AC shallows, the CCC tear will have a greater tendency to move peripherally. Conversely, the deeper the AC, the flatter the anterior lens capsule and therefore the lower the likelihood of the CCC moving posteriorly. The trick is to keep the AC deep and full with viscoelastic. An associated problem is that if the capsulorhexis instrument is not carefully pivoted in the wound, there will be a distortion of the cornea worsening the view. It will also have a knock-on effect by increasing the rate of viscoelastic escaping, so shallowing the AC.

There will also be a greater tendency for the CCC to move peripherally if the flap is torn when not folded over. Always try and keep the flap 'on its back'.

The torn edge has a habit of obscuring the view. This can be elegantly minimised by placing the freshly torn edge in the centre of the eye before releasing it and regrasping the capsule edge nearest the intact capsule.

5. Hydrodissection

This is designed to separate the lens away from the capsule to allow it to spin easily in the capsular bag; it is rather like adding milk around a bowl of porridge. If you watch carefully, you will be able to see the wave-front of the fluid moving across the red reflex; you need to be able to see this in order to judge how much fluid is enough. There are again several different techniques, but they have some common problems.

- Inserting the cannula just under the edge of the capsulorhexis by about 1–2 mm and applying a short smooth injection of BSS should produce a wave-front. After each attempt, there will be a quantity of fluid behind the lens, which should be released; this can be done by gently rocking the nucleus with the cannula while applying a *small* amount of posterior pressure. If this is not done, then repeated attempts will produce a large pocket of posterior fluid, which can potentially rupture the posterior capsule.

- It is often difficult to gauge the exact amount of fluid required, but two injections at 45° to the main axis will usually suffice.

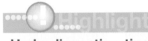

Highlight

Hydrodissection tips

The main difficulty with hydrodissection is gaining the correct amount of pressure with the syringe to produce a good wave-front without rupturing the posterior capsule. As a beginner, the placement of the cannula on the lens prevents subtle anterior movements if the lens induced by hydrodissection injection. It does help considerably to insert the cannula slightly to one side and ensure the more proximal part of the cannula is not lying across the lens, holding it back.

If the nucleus does not easily rotate during phacoemulsification, do not be afraid to try further hydrodissection injections.

6. Phacoemulsification ('phaco')

People have written entire books on this subject (see 'Further reading', p. 286). There are several basic techniques, which will be discussed here along with a few tips for improved success.

The aim of phacoemulsification is to safely remove the nuclear material with as little stress on the zonules as possible. A two-handed technique is now most widespread in use and a variety of second instruments (for the non-dominant hand) are available, e.g. chopper, mushroom etc. (see Ch. 48, 'Surgical instruments'). These are used to assist in the manipulation of the nuclear fragments and cracking the nucleus, once an adequate groove depth has been achieved. They are also useful in the later parts of phaco to place underneath the phaco tip to prevent the posterior capsule from moving up to the phaco tip, this is most crucial at the time of removal of the last nuclear fragment.

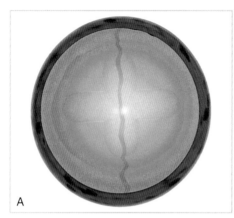
A

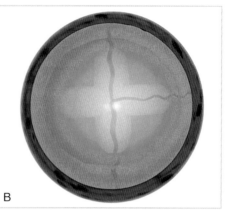
B

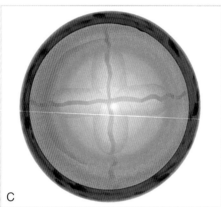
C

Fig. 44.5 Phacoemulsification. A. Once the capsulorhexis is complete the cataract is emulsified with the phaco probe. The technique showed here is referred to as *divide and conquer* and consists of making two perpendicular grooves through about 80% of the depth of the cataract. The nucleus is then cracked through one of the grooves. **B & C.** The cataract is then cracked along each of the remaining grooves, creating four quadrants, which may then be sequentially removed with the phaco probe.

Examples of some of the commoner phaco techniques include the following:

- *Divide and conquer.* This is the commonest starting technique and involves making an initial groove in the nucleus and two side grooves at 90° to allow the nucleus to be broken into four quarters, which are then removed separately (Fig. 44.5).
- *Stop chop (phaco-chop).* This technique involves making an initial groove; the nucleus is then split and each half is then further divided into thirds using a chopping technique to allow removal. Chopping involves placing an instrument between the capsule and the lens nucleus and pulling it towards the phaco tip (already embedded in another part of the lens) to split the lens. It is like a slow and controlled version of wood splitting.
- *Pure chopping (direct chop).* This does not require an initial groove. The phaco tip is buried into the lens nucleus and, using high vacuum settings, is held while the lens is split using the chopping technique. This is not for the faint-hearted and is certainly for more advanced phaco surgeons.

7. Irrigation and aspiration (I&A)

Once the nucleus and cortex have been removed, a residual lining of soft lens material (SLM) remains within the capsular bag; this is removed using I&A. The instruments that are used vary, but the principle remains the same. A high vacuum aspiration probe is used to remove the remnants, while fluid is continuously irrigated into the eye. The probes have a small aspiration port, which allows increased vacuum but lower fluid flow. This results in a more stable anterior chamber.

- The original manual Simcoe is a two-handed device, where the aspiration is generated by the non-dominant hand pulling on the plunger of usually a 5 ml syringe. The Simcoe itself has both an aspiration port and an irrigation port on the end of the tip, usually orientated at 90° to each other.
- Automated I&A hand-pieces are available in which the phaco machine generates the vacuum, which is controlled by the foot pedal. Bimanual I&A ('split bits') is also available, which allows isolated irrigation and aspiration through different instruments.

The most difficult part of I&A is getting to the SLM underneath the main incision. Several automated I&A probes have different interchangeable tips and it may be easier to access some of the material by using a right-angled tip ('90'). Using the manual Simcoe it may be possible to use a different incision, such as the second instrument port, or it may be necessary to make a further paracentesis (e.g. opposite the main incision to access the subincisional SLM).

 Highlight

I&A tips

It is sometimes difficult to remove a section of the SLM without catching the posterior capsule and causing a posterior capsular rupture. If it proves particularly difficult, your options are:

- Asking someone more experienced to remove it.
- Getting at it from another entry point.
- Leaving it in and removing it when the lens is in situ, when the PC will be better protected.
- Nobody will be impressed if you rupture the posterior capsule chasing soft lens matter under the main incision!

8. IOL insertion

The eye will need to be refilled with a viscoelastic in order to maintain its shape for lens insertion. There are several techniques available for lens insertion, with many units still using foldable lenses. If a foldable lens is being used, then the wound will probably have to be enlarged, with the associated undesirable astigmatic effects. If the lens is being injected, this will allow insertion through a smaller incision, but care must be taken to avoid the haptics of the lens causing damage to the posterior capsule. Older style rigid lenses (still used in ECCE surgery) required the wound to be extended to ≈6 mm, which therefore usually required sutures to close the wound.

- *Foldable lenses.* These may be folded for you by the scrub nurse, or you may have to do it yourself. The lenses are all designed so that the haptics, when in the eye, point anticlockwise. The lenses are not symmetrical so it **does** matter which way round they go in! Lens insertion techniques vary considerably, particularly dependent on the type of lens used, so watch someone else carefully and practise in the wet lab if possible.

- *Injectable lenses.* These allow the lens to be inserted through a smaller wound but often require more complex manoeuvres to ensure correct positioning. It is more difficult to visualise the lens as it leaves the injector and a slow and measured approach is needed initially. When the IOL pops straight into the capsular bag, it can be a very satisfying technique. They are, however, often more expensive.

Closing up

This entails removing the viscoelastic, which can be done with the I&A probe. The AC often needs to be reformed using BSS and the wounds checked to ensure that they remain self-sealing. Hydration of the wound can be used as a temporary measure to seal minor leaks, otherwise a 10/0 nylon suture may be needed. Some form of postoperative antibiotic is commonly used, such as a subconjunctival or intracameral injection of a cephalosporin, and many units also use subconjunctival betamethasone to reduce postoperative inflammation.

Writing the notes

Most cataract operations are routine and documenting the completion of the basic stages with a comment to that effect will usually suffice (see Box below). The surgeon, IOL inserted and drugs used will need to be documented, as will follow-up plans and the postoperative drop regimen. It is often helpful to document incision locations and phaco times for future audit purposes and also which machine was used, if different machines are available within the department.

Complications must be recorded in the notes, as should steps which have been taken to minimise their impact on the patient. Incident reporting should also be completed and varies between establishments. The theatre scrub nurse should always know the procedure.

Example

Example of cataract surgical notes

Operation: Surgeon:

Date: Anaesthetic used:

Stages

Wound

Viscoelastic in (& type)

CCC

Hydrodissection

Phaco – e.g. chop   Phaco Power:

I&A   Phaco time:

IOL – location and power

Viscoelastic out

Sutures?

Subconjunctival/intracameral injections

Complications:

Postoperative drop regimen and follow-up:

Cataract surgical equipment

JP Kersey

Types of phaco machine

There are two main types of phaco machine, the difference being the manner in which the machine generates vacuum for aspiration. While neither machine is specifically better, they do have their differences and recognising these differences will allow you to get the best out of a specific machine.

Venturi machines

This type of machine generates vacuum by blowing compressed air past a small tube. This draws air out of the small tube generating a vacuum. This vacuum is applied to a rigid cassette, which in turn is applied to the tubing connecting to the phaco tip. The cassette needs to be rigid to prevent it from collapsing. If the vacuum rises in the cassette, it does so also at the phaco tip, so increasing the rate of fluid aspiration. The machine can control the vacuum level and so indirectly the aspiration rate.

Peristaltic or rotatory pump machines

These machines use a rotating pump head, which massages fluid along the tubing. The pump lies between the phaco hand-piece and the drainage container, which does not need to be rigid (cf. Venturi machines). The rate of aspiration is dependent on the rate of pump head rotation. If the phaco is occluded, then vacuum is generated. If not occluded, then increasing rotation speed increases the rate of aspiration, not vacuum. Limits on aspiration rate and maximum vacuum can be set independently.

Foot pedals

There are two foot pedals used in phaco. The microscope pedal is more commonly used under the left foot and controls zoom, focus, X-Y control and on/off for the microscope light.

Microscope pedal

There are of course variations, but most pedals will have an on/off button for the microscope light and a joystick for control of the field of view in the X-Y control. There are usually two other control pedals, which are often of the rocker variety. One will control zoom and the other focus. Make sure that the X-Y controls and the focus controls are in the middle of their ranges before starting each case; this often necessitates pressing a single button on the side of the microscope. It is considerably more difficult to alter once you have started.

Phaco pedal

The phaco machine foot pedal (Figs 45.1 and 45.2) can be programmed for many functions, but the basic functions are to control the irrigation, vacuum and phaco power (ultrasound) used. On some machines, there are two different settings for the phaco pedal, the easiest to learn being linear:

- *Linear.* The first part of the foot pedal depression activates the irrigation. The second stage of travel initiates aspiration or vacuum. This increases with the level of depression in a linear fashion. Once you reach the end of the second stage, the ultrasound (phaco power) will start and will increase linearly with further depression until the pedal is fully depressed. At this point, the machine will be producing maximum aspiration and maximum phaco power. In this set-up it is only possible to have phaco power if you have maximum vacuum/aspiration.
- *Dual linear.* This allows the phaco power and vacuum to be controlled independently. There are only two stages to the depression of the pedal,

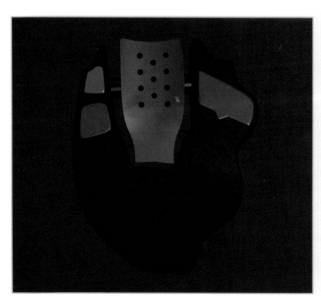

Fig. 45.1 Phaco pedal.
This is an example of a pedal used to control the phacoemulsification process. In this model, the pedal is able to yaw from side to side to control the phaco power (useful in dual linear phacoemulsification), as well as vertical movements to control the aspiration independently.

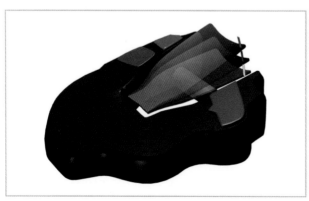

Fig. 45.2 Operation of phaco pedal. Movement of the pedal in the vertical plane will allow the operator to switch on irrigation alone (1), irrigation and aspiration (2) or irrigation, aspiration and phacoemulsification (3).

initially irrigation and then aspiration. The phaco power is independently controlled with a yaw movement (turning the foot to the side).

As dual linear control adds further things to think about, it is likely that inexperienced surgeons will start with a straight linear control.

Types of intraocular lenses (IOL)

Advances in intraocular lenses have come a long way since Sir Harold Ridley's discovery of the inert nature of Perspex fragments in aircraft pilots' eyes.
Modern lenses can be classified as follows:

- *Material.* Lens materials include silicone (which is now in its fourth generation), HMMA, PMMA and acrylic types. Lens material can have a dramatic effect on the rate of posterior capsular opacification and so most companies now produce lenses which aim to reduce this.
- *Hydrophilic vs. hydrophobic.* The underlying IOL molecule (e.g. silicone) is then altered to make it hydrophilic or hydrophobic. This can affect the choice of lens, as some surgeons feel happier using a specific type of material. Hydrophobic lenses may be safer in children, as they are less likely to uptake water during the long time that they will remain within the eye.
- *Shape.* The lens shape can also reduce posterior capsular opacification; a square edge to the lens is now often the preferred option with most surgeons. The square edge can cause a glinting effect known as the 'edge effect' and efforts to reduce this by making a frosted square edge have been used.
- *Coatings.* Lenses can be coated with heparin, which has been shown to have some effect in reducing postoperative inflammation. These are used in eyes that may have a high risk of postoperative uveitis.
- *Monofocal, multifocal or accommodative.* Most IOLs used in public hospitals are of the fixed focus, monofocal design. Others, which are used predominantly in the private sector, include:

  - Multifocal lenses: these lenses are multifocal, with zones of varying refractive power. Patients have to learn to ignore images produced by different areas of the lens while looking at either close or distant objects. Patients sometimes have problems with absolute visual acuity, or glare while night driving, which can reduce the level of satisfaction following surgery.

  - Flexible accommodative lenses: these lenses are designed to move within the eye. Accommodative effort induces contraction of the ciliary body, which exerts pressure on the vitreous body, which in turn displaces the IOL forward a small distance. In some eyes this may be enough to produce reading vision.

  - Other types of lens: various experimental lenses exist, which work by refilling the capsular bag with a polymeric substance. Such lenses offer the possible future prospect of restoring accommodation completely.

Spotting the difficult cataract

JP Kersey

The following are examples of potentially difficult situations in cataract surgery, where either precautions must be taken prior to surgery or an experienced surgeon should perform the case.

Dense white cataract with no fundal view

B scan ultrasonography may be needed to exclude gross fundal pathology, which may contraindicate surgery (e.g. a choroidal tumour or chronic retinal detachment). Checking for an RAPD prior to pupillary dilatation is a good way of spotting advanced retinal pathology, but will not exclude macular disease. Visualisation of the capsulorhexis will be difficult, and vision blue may be needed.

Extreme refractive error

Most departments stock a good range of IOLs; however, this usually only spans 15 to 30 D. If you need an IOL outside this range, it is worth checking with the theatre staff as early as possible (e.g. at the time of preassessment).

High myopia
These patients often have large eyes and very floppy posterior capsules, particularly at the time of removal of the last nuclear fragment. Care must be taken not to phaco the posterior capsule.

High hypermetropia
These patients have small eyes and often shallow ACs, which reduces the space to operate until adequate room has been made by the removal of the first nuclear fragment.

Pseudoexfoliation syndrome

These patients are likely to have very loose zonules and must be treated very carefully, often by increasing phaco power and ensuring that only absolutely necessary movements are made. Insertion of a capsular tension ring may help to increase the stability.

Common ophthalmic surgical procedures

Previous Trabeculectomy

These patients are likely to be operated on by the glaucoma team and are at risk of postoperative inflammation, which may induce bleb failure. They may require a subconjunctival 5 FU (5 fluorouracil) injection near the bleb after surgery. This may need to be ordered, so check with the theatre staff.

The small pupil

These eyes present a problem because the small pupil not only considerably reduces the view, but also the working space in the centre of the eye. It prevents adequate visualisation of the nuclear fragments and soft lens matter, increasing the risk of incomplete removal of these elements. The pupil can be stretched using a variety of techniques but this may tear the iris, which can then bleed; it will also become floppier, increasing its tendency to prolapse into the phaco port. Iris hooks may be used to hold the iris back, but their use requires guidance and careful placement.

Fuch's endothelial dystrophy

These eyes have a very low endothelial cell count and are at risk of developing corneal cloudiness midway through and after the procedure. Minimising phaco power and fragment manipulation, as well as using a coating viscoelastic, will help to reduce endothelial cell loss.

Phacodonesis/iridodonesis

The spontaneous wobbling of a lens or iris at the slitlamp implies loose zonules; it may be seen, for example, in the setting of pseudoexfoliation syndrome (see above) or a traumatic cataract. A tension ring is often a prerequisite for successful surgery.

Blepharitis

If advanced or particularly purulent, blepharitis represents a contraindication to surgery until treated.

General issues

- *Deep set eyes.* Such eyes can be very difficult in terms of access and should not be attempted by junior surgeons.
- *Phimotic eyelids.* As above.
- *'Squeezers'.* Some patients, even with a good anaesthetic, are able to cause considerable difficulty for the surgeon through contraction of the orbicularis

oculi muscle. If there is difficulty, for example, when checking the intraocular pressure, bear in mind that surgery may be difficult.

- *Tremor.* Consider general anaesthesia.

- *Mental health issues.* Consider general anaesthesia.

- *Posture.* Some patients are unable to lie flat; such situations are best dealt with by an experienced surgeon.

- *Patients with chronic obstructive pulmonary disease.* These patients may need a very low operation time to minimise their respiratory discomfort. In addition, they often produce a large amount of positive vitreous pressure, which can lead to challenging surgical conditions and very shallow ACs.

- *First eye complications.* If the first eye's operation was complicated, it is highly likely that there may also be an inherent problem in the ocular anatomy of the second eye. Proceed carefully.

- *Drugs.* Recently, it has been noticed that patients taking tamsulosin for prostatic/urinary problems are at a greatly increased risk of the intraoperative floppy iris syndrome. Appropriate precautions, such as the use of iris hooks, should be considered.

Anaesthesia for ocular surgery

JP Kersey

Introduction

There are many ways of establishing effective ocular anaesthesia. In cataract surgery, the technique favoured in many units is often down to the personal preference of the individual surgeons.

Topical anaesthesia

This is increasingly becoming the preferred anaesthetic technique for the experienced cataract surgeon and is often used in conjunction with an intra-cameral injection of anaesthetic. It removes the risk of globe penetration associated with sharp needle techniques, but it has a short duration of action and is not usually adequate if anterior vitrectomy is needed. The patient can also move the eye, which requires a good level of cooperation, especially at delicate parts of the operation such as the capsulorhexis (Ch. 44). Once the phaco probe per se is within the eye, patient movement becomes much less of a problem.

Postoperative visual recovery is much quicker than with other forms of anaesthesia.

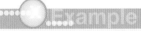

Example

Types of anaesthetic drop commonly used

- Tetracaine (amethocaine)—longest lasting, can cause cornea clouding.
- Benoxinate.
- Proxymetacaine (least unpleasant for patient, shortest acting).

Sub-Tenon's anaesthesia

This is an excellent form of anaesthesia if performed well, although it is a technique that takes some mastering to get reliable results. Poor technique can lead to a lack of akinesia and occasionally marked chemosis, which can lead to pooling of the irrigating fluid, so reducing the view.

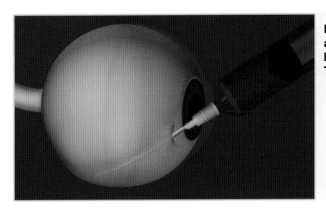

Fig. 47.1 A sub-Tenon's anaesthetic is placed between the sclera and Tenon's capsule.

This technique uses a gently curved, blunt cannula, which is inserted through an incision made in the conjunctiva and Tenon's layers. The cannula is slid along the surface of the sclera to the peribulbar space where the local anaesthetic is injected (Fig. 47.1). Once in the correct plane, tilting the syringe to the vertical position allows the best location for injection. The anaesthetic agents used often include a shorter acting local anaesthetic mixed with a longer acting agent, such as bupivacaine. These agents are often mixed with hyaluronidase, which acts to break down some of the fibrous attachments in this space and aids spread of the agents, so improving the nature of the block. The technique does not involve the use of a sharp needle and so greatly reduces the risk of globe perforation, although this has still been reported.

The drawbacks are that there is a considerable learning curve to master the technique, it can cause marked subconjunctival haemorrhages and there is a risk of temporary postoperative diplopia, as akinesia is induced.

Peribulbar anaesthesia

This is still the preferred technique in some centres, though it is becoming less common for cataract surgery. However, if it is anticipated that the procedure may be prolonged or is at a high risk of needing an anterior vitrectomy, then a peribulbar anaesthetic would ensure that the eye would already be prepared. It is still a reliable technique for procedures that may require deeper levels of anaesthesia for longer periods (such as trabeculectomy), producing excellent levels of anaesthesia. Substantial akinesia is easily induced, but as a result this does reduce the level of resistance available (if you move your instrument, you will move the eye).

A sharp needle, often 25 G, is inserted beneath the globe at the intersection between the lateral third and medial two-thirds of the orbital rim (Fig. 47.2). This can be done through the skin or, more commonly, the conjunctiva. The needle is then passed around the globe to the peribulbar space where the local anaesthetic agents are injected (Fig. 47.3). A mixture of short- and long-acting anaesthetic agents and hyaluronidase are usually used (see above, as per sub-Tenon's anaesthesia).

Common ophthalmic surgical procedures

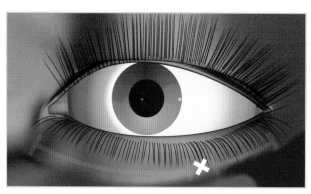

Fig. 47.2 A peribulbar anaesthetic can be given though the lower lid skin or through an anaesthetised conjunctiva. The landmark is shown here with a white cross.

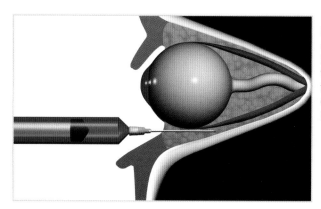

Fig. 47.3 Peribulbar anaesthesia. The needle is inserted to a point behind the equator of the eye and the anaesthetic injected outside the muscle cone (peribulbar).

This technique carries a definite risk of retrobulbar haemorrhage and globe perforation, both of which can lead to a permanent loss of vision. Postoperative visual recovery can be delayed by several hours and usually includes a period of diplopia. Other side-effects include chemosis and temporarily reduced visual acuity.

Retrobulbar anaesthesia

This is now a less commonly used technique and has been discredited for its increased rate of ocular perforation. Some surgeons/anaesthetists use a longer needle to perform a peribulbar anaesthetic and often enter the muscle cone behind the globe (i.e. a retrobulbar anaesthetic). This considerably improves the akinetic effect of the anaesthetic but has a notable higher risk of globe perforation. The College do not recommend this as a routine anaesthetic technique.

Highlight

Tips and pitfalls in ocular local anaesthesia

- The bevel of the needle placed facing the globe will reduce the risk of perforation.

- Hyaluronidase can induce orbital inflammation, particularly in higher concentrations.

- Sub-Tenon's anaesthetic needs to be placed as posteriorly as possible to reduce chemosis.

General anaesthesia (GA)

This is now infrequently used, as day-case surgery has taken hold and people are becoming increasingly confident in the use of topical and regional anaesthesia. Patients admitted for surgery under GA add an extra dimension, as they must be assessed for their fitness for the anaesthetic, as well as necessitating a hospital bed. Increasingly, GA is being reserved for young patients, those for whom cooperation during the operation would be difficult, and when requested by the patient.

Surgical instruments

MJ Hawker

'Give us the tools and we will finish the job.'
Winston Churchill, 1941

Introduction

The subject of ophthalmic instruments is large enough to justify a textbook in its own right. Instrument design, intended use, technique, care and sterilisation are all important aspects. When starting a surgical apprenticeship, developing an understanding of the 'tools of the job' that will enable best surgical performance is essential. Successful use of instruments in a surgical procedure involves a mixture of the specific design and intended use of an instrument for a specific purpose, together with the personalised surgical idiosyncrasies that come only with experience. Whilst this chapter cannot offer the latter, an overview of the former with regard to the major ophthalmic procedures is an important starting point.

Due to limitations of space, the chapter will concentrate on those instruments in common use, to help the reader recognise each by name and to understand each instrument's proper use. Images included in this chapter are taken (with permission) from the Duckworth and Kent catalogue (manufacturers of titanium precision surgical instruments; see 'Useful contacts', p. 287). Where instrument names are specific to this catalogue, the more familiar name is included in parentheses.

Cataract surgery

The eyelids are held open by a speculum (Fig. 48.1). Specula can be of single piece construction, adjustable, angled to rest temporally or nasally (ease of access for temporal surgery), and optionally with solid blades to keep eyelashes away from the surgical field. Open blades are commonly used because they interfere less with other instruments.

Corneal incisions are performed using keratomes to create the initial corneal or limbal groove and side-port incisions (Fig. 48.2). If three-step incisions are planned, the second step is usually performed using a crescent blade. The anterior chamber is then entered using the spear-shaped keratome to create a wound of known width, which will allow entry of the phacoemulsification probe tip.

During the placement of incisions, the globe is stabilised by holding the conjunctiva with minimally traumatic forceps (a variety are available), or by using a Thornton's ring (Fig. 48.3). In order to grasp tissues, forceps are toothed

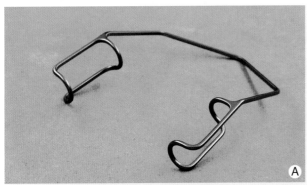

Fig. 48.1 Speculum.
A. Barraquer adult speculum. **B.** Barrett adjustable speculum. (All images in this chapter courtesy of Duckworth & Kent Ltd: Titanium Surgical Instruments.)

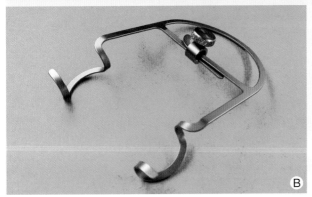

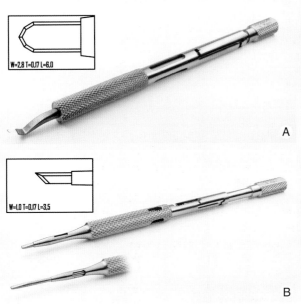

Fig. 48.2 Instruments for corneal incisions.
A. Pearce angled retractable diamond knife 2.8 mm.
B. Pearce 45° retractable diamond knife.

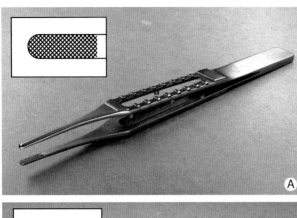

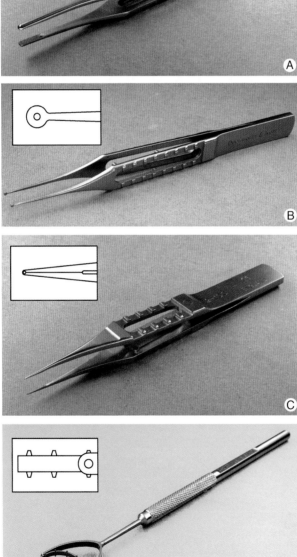

Fig. 48.3 Instruments used to stabilise globe during cataract surgery.
A. Moorfields forceps (in titanium). **B.** Osher conjunctival forceps.
C. Pierse notched forceps.
D. Thornton fixation ring.

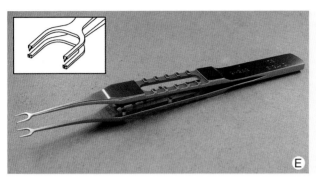

Fig. 48.3 (cont'd) E. Bores corneal fixation forceps.

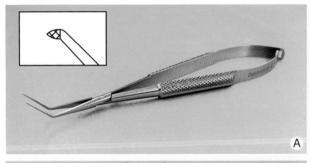

Fig. 48.4 Capsulorhexis and hydrodissection instruments. A. Utrata capsulorhexis forceps. **B.** Mackool hydrodissection cannula.

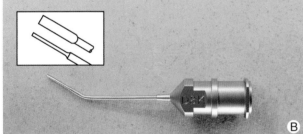

(can be traumatic) or notched (less traumatic). Double fixation forceps are also available to provide two points of fixation to prevent rotation of the globe. Forceps generally come with different designs of handle to allow different techniques suitable for varying surgical situations. The tips of forceps may have tying platforms incorporated to allow suture manipulation.

The capsulorhexis is usually started with an insulin syringe needle bent to the surgeon's preference, or a preformed cystotome (Fig. 48.4). Capsulorhexis forceps are often used to complete the manoeuvre. Hydrodissection is then performed, for which a variety of cannulae are available. A 'J' shaped cannula ensures sufficient hydrodissection under the corneal wound.

During phacoemulsification, various 'second instruments' can be used via the side-port incision to manipulate the nucleus (Fig. 48.5). 'Chopping' refers to the use of an instrument to break the nucleus into pieces using the phaco tip as a platform. The major advantage of this technique lies in the lower overall phaco energy required.

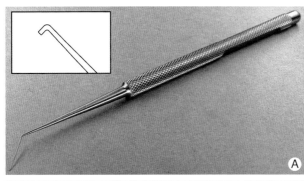

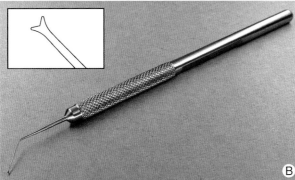

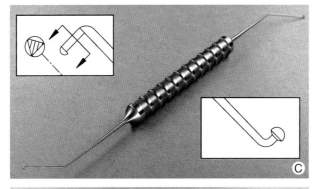

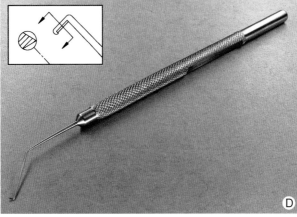

Fig. 48.5 'Second instruments' used during phacoemulsification.
A. Sinskey hook. **B.** Bechert nucleus rotator. **C.** Barrett Duo nucleus rotator/manipulator/splitter. **D.** Nucleus divider (Nagahara chopper).

The intraocular lens is then folded and inserted using specific forceps (Fig. 48.6), or injected. A lens dialler may be used to dial in the trailing haptic. If corneal sutures are required, further instruments are necessary (Fig. 48.7). Needle holders can be straight, curved, and with or without a locking mechanism; most come with round handles for ease of manipulation. Tying forceps have platforms incorporated to grip the suture.

If extracapsular surgery is performed then additional instruments are required (Fig. 48.8). Corneal scissors may be used to complete the initial corneal incision; these are curved to suit either right- or left-handed surgeons. Additionally, a nucleus expressor and lens loop (vectis) are generally used to help express the lens nucleus. Following aspiration of soft lens matter, completion of the capsulorhexis can be performed using capsule scissors.

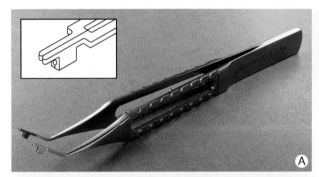

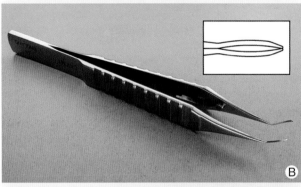

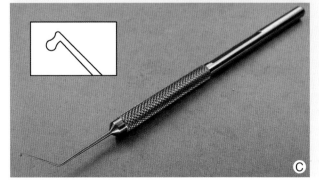

Fig. 48.6 Specialised forceps for folding and inserting the intraocular lens. A. IOL folding forceps. **B.** IOL insertion forceps, with lock. **C.** O'Gawa standard IOL dialler.

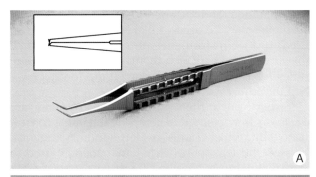
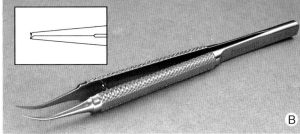

Fig. 48.7 Forceps for corneal suturing. A. Kelman McPherson suturing forceps. **B.** Nordan suturing forceps.

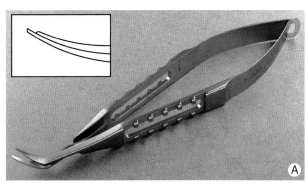
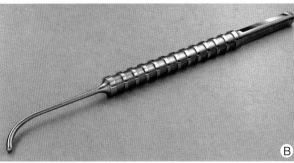

Fig. 48.8 Extracapsular surgical instruments. A. Castroviejo corneal scissors (curved to right). **B.** Barrett nucleus expressor.

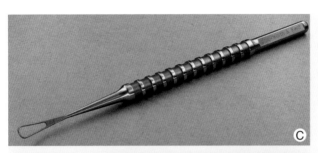

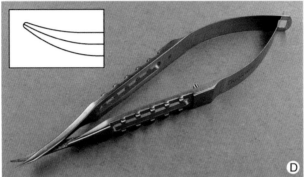

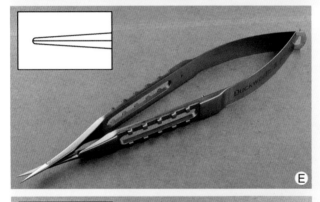

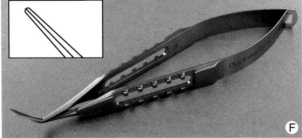

Fig. 48.8 (cont'd)
C. Barrett modified lens loop. **D.** Capsule scissors (curved). **E.** Vannas scissors (straight). **F.** Gills Vannas scissors (Ong's).

Minor lid procedures

Instruments used for minor lid procedures are shown in Figures 48.9 and 48.10. When removing chalazia, a chalazion clamp is used to evert the lid, prevent bleeding and provide a platform for curettage. Different sized chalazion clamps and curettes are available. Specific forceps are available for epilation. If required, double eversion of the upper lid is performed using the Desmarres lid retractor. Punctal dilators are designed to dilate the punctum to allow the passage of lacrimal probes. Specific toothed forceps are available to handle the lid tissues during oculoplastic procedures.

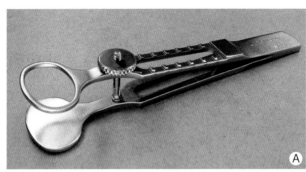

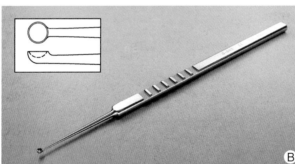

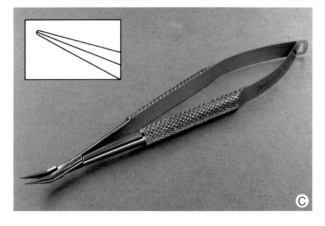

Fig. 48.9 Instruments used for minor lid procedures. A. Desmarres chalazion forceps/clamp. **B.** Meyerhoefer chalazion curette. **C.** Kudo cilia forceps.

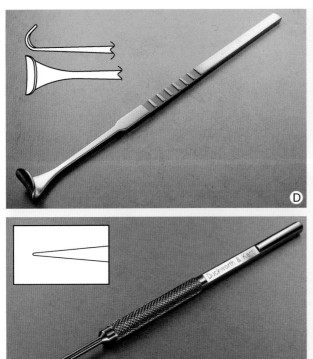

D

E

Fig. 48.9 (cont'd)
D. Desmarres lid retractor.
E. Lacrimal dilator.

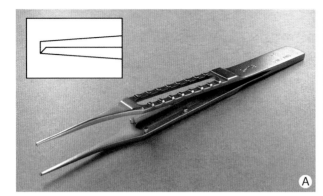

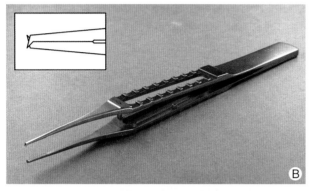

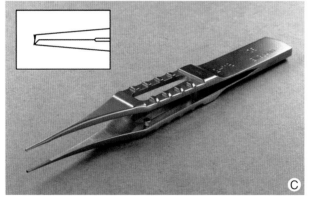

Fig. 48.10 Toothed forceps for handling lid tissue during procedures.
A. Rabkin blepharoplasty tissue forceps (Jales).
B. Castroviejo suturing forceps (Listers). **C.** Bonn suturing forceps (St Martin's).

Squint surgery

During extraocular muscle surgery, muscle hooks are used to isolate the required muscles (Fig. 48.11). The Jameson hook spreads the muscle fibres out to allow accurate suture placement. The exact length of muscle requiring resection or recession is measured using callipers. Tenotomy scissors are then used to cut the muscle.

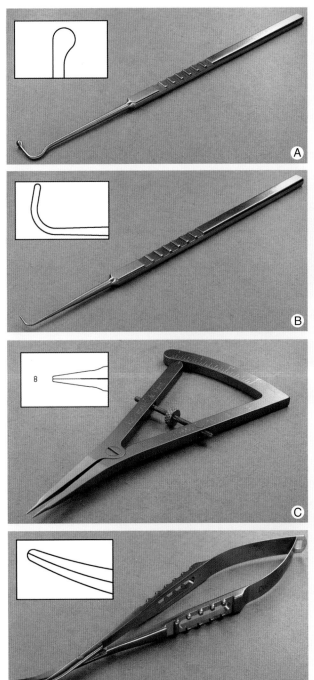

Fig. 48.11 Instruments used in squint surgery.
A. Jameson muscle hook. **B.** Paediatric muscle hook. **C.** Castroviejo style marking calliper. **D.** Westcott style tenotomy scissors (curved).

Common ophthalmic surgical procedures

Surgical correction of astigmatism

During cataract surgery, it is sometimes desirable to perform corneal incisions in the treatment of astigmatism (Fig. 48.12; see also Ch. 4). Relaxing incisions are placed on the steep meridian of corneal curvature with a length and depth that varies according to corneal position, patient age and degree of astigmatism (nomograms are available to guide the surgeon). During the placement of limbal or corneal relaxing incisions, the direction of the steep axis is confirmed using a

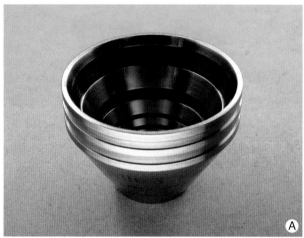

A

Fig. 48.12 Instruments used in surgical correction of astigmatism. A. Maloney keratometer. **B.** Mendez degree gauge. **C.** Thornton arcuate guarded diamond knife.

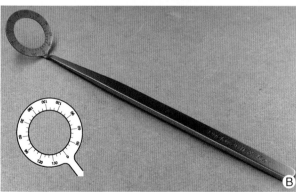

B

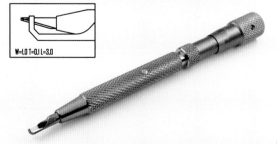

C

handheld keratometer. Viewed under the operating microscope, the reflection shape of the concentric rings depends on the degree and axis of astigmatism. A degree gauge is used to mark the position of the steep axis (measured preoperatively using keratometry and corneal topography) and to mark the length of intended incisions. The incisions are then performed using guarded blades of preset depth.

49

Ophthalmic therapeutic lasers

JP Kersey

Note: The settings suggested in this chapter are for guidance only. Laser machines vary widely and local colleagues should be consulted to find the ideal settings for a particular machine. Operation of lasers should be in accordance with local policy and protocol regarding safety. Protective goggles should be worn by observers at all times.

Nd:YAG (neodymium: yttrium aluminium garnet) laser

Nd:YAG capsulotomy

This procedure uses a Nd:YAG ('YAG') laser to create a hole in the posterior capsule following the development of posterior capsular opacification (PCO, Fig. 49.1). The YAG laser is usually mounted onto a slitlamp to allow the patient's head to be fixed using the chin and forehead rests. It uses a laser of 1024 nm wavelength, which is in the infrared spectrum and therefore requires a visible aiming beam, usually a helium:neon laser (He:Ne beam). The laser is focused by bringing the two (or sometimes four) aiming points together (Fig. 49.2). This is usually performed by focusing beyond the capsule then pulling the joystick back towards yourself to bring the beams together to a point.

Firing the laser makes a small hole in the capsule. A further small hole is made next to it, then another small hole and so on, so forming a line across the capsule. There are several different methods of producing the required hole in the capsule. The line of small holes can be made to form a paracentric ring (Fig. 49.3), and the disc of capsule is then pushed back into the vitreous. Alternatively, a cruciate pattern creates flaps, which can be pushed out of the way (Fig. 49.4). This latter technique has recently been shown to generally require less laser shots (and therefore energy).

There is often an additional control to allow the laser to be defocused, i.e. the Nd:YAG beam will fire beyond the aiming beam by a preset amount; this allows the IOL to be protected (to a degree) from lens laser pits.

Example

YAG capsulotomy: suggested settings

- Start with a 0.8 mJ single shot.
- Increase the power with thicker capsules.
- Adjust defocus if required.

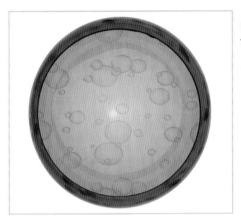

Fig. 49.1 Posterior capsule opacity in the form of Elschnig's pearls.

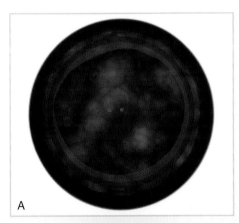

A

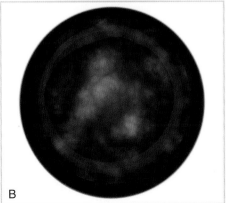

B

Fig. 49.2 Focusing the YAG laser.
A. If two aiming beam dots are seen on the posterior capsule, the laser is focused either too anteriorly (will cause lens pits) or too posteriorly (energy will be dissipated into the vitreous cavity). **B.** One dot will be seen when the two aiming beam dots are brought together to focus the laser on the posterior capsule.

Common ophthalmic surgical procedures

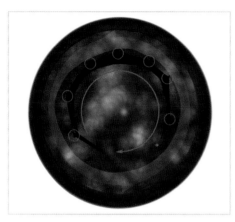

Fig. 49.3 YAG capsulotomy involves clearing the opaque posterior capsule from the visual axis. This diagram illustrates a circular pattern, starting at 8 o'clock and moving clockwise. Each red ring indicates where shots were fired at the capsule. The red dot shows the laser in focus on the posterior capsule.

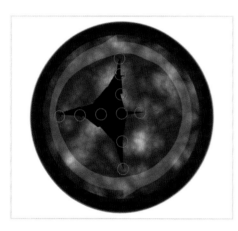

Fig. 49.4 A cross is often made in the posterior capsule instead of a circle. The corners created in the centre tend to fold back out of the visual axis.

Consent

- The procedure usually requires the use of a contact lens that will be removed after the procedure.

- Complications include:

  - Cystoid macular oedema.

  - Pressure spikes—partially prevented by preoperative topical apraclonidine.

  - Lens pits can occur but usually do not affect vision, though several can cause glare.

  - Retinal detachment (very rare).

Nd:YAG iridotomy

This procedure uses a YAG laser to create a hole in the peripheral iris to allow an alternative pathway for aqueous movement in narrow angle and pupillary block glaucoma. The laser is focused in a crypt of the iris and an initial hole is made which is then enlarged. A full thickness hole is appreciated by the appearance of a pigment gush through the iridotomy and a change in shape of the anterior chamber can often be appreciated.

From a medicolegal perspective, it is important to compare the gonioscopic appearance of the angle before and after the iridotomy to ensure that treatment has been successful.

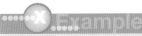

YAG iridotomy: suggested settings

- 4 mJ double pulsed shot initially.
- Then 1mJ to enlarge.

Consent
- The procedure requires the use of a contact lens (e.g. Abrahams type).
- Complications include:
  - Pressure spikes.
  - Cataract (rare).
  - Bleeding of an iris vessel can obscure the view and may delay completing the procedure—preoperative topical apraclonidine reduces the risk of bleeding. (Pressure on the contact lens will usually stop any bleeding during the procedure.)
  - The iridotomy can seal up at a later date requiring a repeat procedure.

Nd:YAG vitreous strand lysis (anterior vitreolysis)

If a vitreous strand presents to one of the wounds following complicated cataract surgery, it may be possible to use the YAG laser to cut it in vivo.

Argon laser

The argon laser can be delivered via a slitlamp or an indirect ophthalmoscope (and a condensing lens, e.g. 20 D). The latter technique is often used for performing panretinal photocoagulation (PRP) under general anaesthetic.

Pan retinal photocoagulation (PRP)

PRP (Fig. 49.5) is used to prevent and control retinal, iris and trabecular neovascularisation in a number of conditions. It is most commonly used for proliferative diabetic retinopathy. Destruction of the outer retina occurs as the laser energy is absorbed by the retinal pigment epithelium and converted to thermal energy, causing protein coagulation and disruption of the cells within that area. The inner nerve fibre layer is hopefully spared. Despite the widespread use of the argon laser, it is not clear exactly how neovascularisation is so effectively treated by this technique.

Argon laser can produce different wavelengths but the blue/green laser is the commonest used. When performed at the slitlamp, the procedure requires the use of a fundus contact lens to visualise and focus the laser. There are many different styles of lens and it is worth becoming familiar with those available

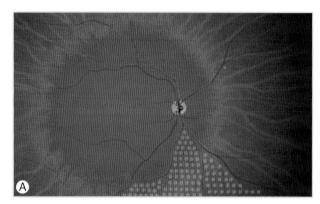

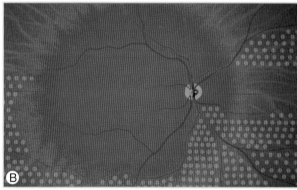

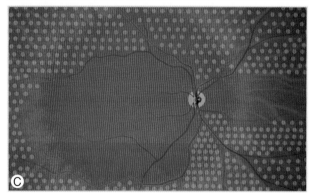

Fig. 49.5 Panretinal photocoagulation (PRP).
A. This procedure involves treating the peripheral retina with evenly spaced laser burns, in this case starting between the inferior arcades. **B.** In the first few PRP treatments, care is taken not to treat the horizontal corridor of nasal retina as this is likely to affect peripheral vision and therefore ability to drive. **C.** Completed first full PRP treatment (with nasal horizontal corridor of retina spared in this case).

locally; they differ in the size of visual field and the degree of magnification, which in turn alter the effective spot size of the laser and so the power needed to produce the desired effect. Such lenses usually have an antireflective coating to minimise the risk to the operator. There is usually a repeat facility on the laser that allows continuous pulsed firing of the beam at a set rate.

There is some discussion as to whether the required endpoint in PRP is a slight whitening of the retina, or a laser burn that is not initially visible. The laser burn will increase in intensity and size around ten minutes after application.

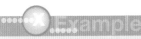

Example

Panretinal photocoagulation (and retinopexy): suggested settings

- Spot size 200–500 µm.
- Duration 0.1 s initially.
- Power initially 100 mW, increase until slight whitening (300–500 mW often necessary).
- Consider using the repeat facility.

Consent

- The procedure can be uncomfortable, especially over the ciliary nerves (3 and 9 o'clock) and local anaesthesia is often used.
- It requires the use of a contact lens, which will be removed after the procedure.
- The eye will be dazzled for ≈30 minutes after the treatment.
- There will be bright flashing lights during the treatment.
- Stress the importance of keeping the eye still.
- Not to look at the He:Ne aiming beam (red light).
- The laser is designed to arrest further deterioration, not improve vision.
- The vision may decline despite laser.
- Further treatments may be necessary.
- It is possible that the patient's ability to drive will be compromised as a result of visual field loss after particularly heavy or multiple treatments.

Argon macular laser

This uses argon laser to reduce oedema and retinal thickening close to the fovea. The indications for macular laser are diabetic macular oedema as set out by the ETDRS trial, and oedema associated with branch retinal vein occlusions, as set out by the branch vein occlusion study. Other indications are the treatment of extrafoveal subretinal neovascular membranes and leaking macroaneurysms.

The procedure requires the use of a contact lens and has similar concerns as PRP. However, as the laser is being fired closer to the fovea, particular emphasis must be made of the importance of the eye remaining still and not looking at the aiming beam. In addition, because the targets for laser are so close to fixation, paracentral scotomata may be appreciated by the patient after the procedure and patients must be warned of this before treatment.

The power required is often lower (start around 50–80 mW), and the number of laser shots used is considerably less than with PRP. A smaller spot size (50–100 µm) is typically used. Due to the presence of blue light-absorbing xanthophyll pigment in the macular neuroretina, only argon green (and not blue-green) should be used.

Common ophthalmic surgical procedures

Argon laser retinopexy

This procedure uses the argon laser to ring-fence a retinal break or tear to prevent rhegmatogenous retinal detachment (Fig. 49.6, and Fig. 52.1, p. 228). It uses a contact lens in a similar fashion to PRP (and similar laser settings). It is sometimes difficult with anterior breaks to adequately encircle the anterior aspect of the lesion, in which case indirect laser with indentation or cryotherapy is used. This is obviously best performed by someone experienced in such techniques.

Due to the often peripheral nature of pathology, patients can be asked to look in a particular direction to aid visualisation.

Consent

- The procedure requires the use of a contact lens, which will be removed afterwards.
- The eye will be dazzled for up to 30 minutes after the treatment.
- There will be bright flashing lights during the procedure.
- Importance of keeping eye still, in the direction requested.
- Not to look at the He:Ne aiming beam (red light).
- Retinal detachment may occur despite laser.
- Further treatments may be necessary.
- Pain during procedure.
- Small risk of epiretinal fibrosis (may potentially lead to late loss of sight).

Argon laser trabeculoplasty

This procedure uses the argon laser to cause scarring in the anterior trabecular meshwork. This is thought to act by stretching the posterior meshwork and so increasing the aqueous outflow. The technique is generally felt to have a limited temporal effect, lasting for up to five years, but may be repeated as usually only half the meshwork is treated at any one time. It is a procedure that is more popular in the United States than in Great Britain. The procedure is performed using a gonioscopic contact lens with an antireflective laser coating.

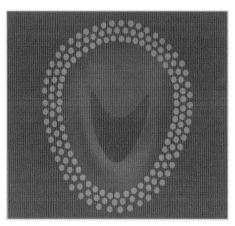

Fig. 49.6 Retinal tear. A U-shaped tear in the retina with a (very small) localised retinal detachment. Three rows of laser burns are placed around the tear. Note that only the surrounding, attached retina is treated.

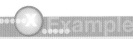

Argon laser trabeculoplasty: suggested settings

Start with 800 mW power (often 1000–1200 mW is necessary), a 0.1 s duration and a spot size of 50 μm. Approximately 15–20 burns are placed in each quarter (3 clock hours) of the anterior trabeculum. Usually, 180–270° of the anterior trabeculum is treated in a single session. The inferior trabeculum is often easier to visualise than the superior.

Argon laser iridoplasty

This is an uncommon procedure, but is performed to treat the plateau iris configuration and associated syndrome. Broad, low-power, long-duration laser burns are placed through 360° of the peripheral iris, causing a contraction and so changing the abnormal configuration of the peripheral iris.

Argon laser iridoplasty: suggested settings

- Power: 200–240 mW.
- Duration: 0.5 s.
- Spot size: 500 μm.
- Full 360° treatment usual.
- Use Abrahams-style iridotomy lens.

Argon suture lysis

Following a trabeculectomy it may be necessary to release one of the sutures placed through the scleral flap and this can be done using the argon laser. The patient's eye is anaesthetised using topical anaesthetic and the suture is lasered, often using a contact lens similar to that used for peripheral iridotomy (Zeiss type four-mirror lens also often used). Argon suture stretch has also been performed (although less commonly) and involves lasering the suture with a lower power, so producing a gentle warming (and thus stretching) of the suture.

Argon laser suture lysis: suggested settings

- Power: 300 mW (sometimes requiring up to 1000 mW).
- Duration: 0.1 s.
- Spot size: 50 μm.
- Usually only one shot needed.

Diode laser

This laser is used for treating several different conditions including refractory glaucoma, subretinal neovascular membranes and retinal tumours. Its use in neovascular membranes and retinal lesions is complicated by the fact that no visible endpoint is achieved; the power and duration of the treatment must therefore be carefully calculated prior to its use. The settings are dependent primarily on the size of the area being treated and the nature of the lesion.

Cyclodiode treatment

This is the most commonly performed diode laser procedure and is gaining in popularity as a method of controlling high intraocular pressures in patients refractory to topical therapy and unsuitable for surgery, such as patients with neovascular glaucoma. Multiple treatments can be given and are performed under a local anaesthetic block such as peribulbar or sub-Tenon's. In neovascular patients, it can also be used to produce anterior retinal ablation and regression of neovascularisation.

For cyclodestruction, typically 15–20 shots are used, through 9 clock hours (270°) of the ciliary body, often using 2000 mW for 2 seconds per shot. 'Pops' (representing cavitation and destruction within the ciliary body) are often heard and are worth documenting in the notes.

Consent

- The procedure is done to reduce the pressure in the eye by reducing the aqueous production.
- The treatment may not adequately reduce the pressure, so further treatment may be required.
- The treatment could stop aqueous production altogether and lead to phthisis bulbi.
- The vision may worsen after the procedure, but this usually recovers quickly.
- The procedure is not designed to stop the underlying condition.

Further Information

References

- Early Treatment of Diabetic Retinopathy Study Research Group. Photocoagulation for diabetic macular edema. Early Treatment of Diabetic Retinopathy Study report number 1. Arch Ophthalmol 1985; 103 (12): 1796–806.

- The Branch Vein Occlusion Study Group. Argon laser photocoagulation for macular edema in branch vein occlusion. Am J Ophthalmol 1984; 98 (3): 271–82.

- Ritch R, Tham CCY, Lam DSC. Long-term success of argon laser peripheral iridoplasty in the management of the plateau iris syndrome. Ophthalmology 2004; 111(1): 104–8.

- Savage JA, Condon GP, Lytle RA, Simmons RJ. Laser suture lysis after trabeculectomy. Ophthalmology 1988; 95: 1631–8.

50

Trabeculectomy

SN Madge

Introduction

These days, most trainee ophthalmologists will probably not perform a trabeculectomy until at least registrar grade, although in years gone by it was often an operation that was left to the most junior surgeon to complete. There is a vast amount of literature written about the operation, which can be quite daunting for the newcomer to the speciality to grasp.

Indications

Trabeculectomies are most commonly performed in patients with glaucoma who fail to reach target intraocular pressures with medical therapy alone. However, as techniques continue to improve, there is an argument that glaucoma patients should be offered the procedure early in the treatment history in order to provide a life free from eyedrops. In addition, prompt and successful surgery may well be considerably cheaper than years of relatively expensive topical medication.

Basic principles

The idea of the operation is to create an alternative drainage pathway for aqueous humour to leave the eye. In a trabeculectomy, a guarded connection is forged between the anterior chamber and the subconjunctival space, creating a drainage 'bleb'. A partial thickness scleral flap limits the flow out of the eye.

Selection/preassessment of patients

Crucial to the success of the operation is a superior conjunctiva free from scarring. Patients with risk factors for failure of the procedure (e.g. history of uveitis, history of glaucoma topical treatment, black race, etc.) should be considered for an 'augmented' trabeculectomy, where antimetabolites (e.g. 5-fluorouracil or mitomycin-C) are used during the operation to reduce postoperative scarring of the conjunctiva, which is thought to be responsible for many trabeculectomy failures. Up-to-date visual fields (if appropriate) should be available and if fixation is threatened, it is worthwhile documenting central vision with, for example, a Humphrey 10-2 test.

Consent

Although every surgeon will have different complication rates, the following qualitative list of risks covers most eventualities:

- Blindness.
- Infection—for years after the procedure (blebitis, endophthalmitis).
- Failure.
- Further surgical procedures, including bleb-related procedures, such as needling or further antimetabolite injection.
- Cataract.
- Bleed (i.e. suprachoroidal haemorrhage).
- Possible change in spectacle prescription.
- Ongoing dependence on eyedrops to achieve a target pressure.
- The use of an antimetabolite.
- Specifically mention that the operation is not being performed to improve vision, but to attempt to maintain it.

The procedure

The following description is purely designed as a brief introduction to the operation for the new ophthalmologist.

- Asepsis and anaesthesia are assumed.
- The conjunctiva and underlying Tenon's tissue are dissected either from the limbus ('fornix-based' flap, as the flap hinges from the fornix) or from deep in the fornix ('limbus-based' flap).
- Diathermy is applied to the underlying scleral vessels to create an avascular area over the area of the planned partial thickness scleral flap.
- If an augmented procedure is planned, 5FU- or MMC-soaked sponges are often placed in the subconjunctival space for a set period of time (e.g. 3 minutes). Generous irrigation is then applied after the removal of the sponges. An alternative method of application of 5FU is to inject it into the subconjunctival space postoperatively, usually fairly posteriorly.
- A partial thickness scleral flap is created and then the anterior chamber is entered (sclerostomy). A punch is then often used to remove trabecular tissue, thus enlarging the hole created.
- A surgical peripheral iridectomy is then performed which prevents plugging of the sclerostomy site by iris, also reducing the risk of angle closure.
- The scleral flap is then sutured down to the sclera, often employing releasable suture techniques. Such sutures can be removed at a period after surgery to allow increased flow. If releasable techniques are not used, the argon laser may be used to perform postoperative laser suture lysis with a similar effect.

- The conjunctiva is then carefully closed over the scleral trapdoor, and fluorescein is then usually applied, utilising the Seidel test to examine for leaks.
- A combination of intense mydriatic, antibiotic and topical corticosteroid treatment is then standard postoperative treatment, with steroids often being continued for months. The patient's routine topical glaucoma eyedrops are omitted in the operated eye. Acetazolamide is also usually avoided postoperatively because its use can lead to failure of the procedure.

The postoperative period

There is a tremendous amount of variation in postoperative trabeculectomy care and it is important to liaise closely with your consultant if asked to review such patients.

On day one, check at least the following:

- visual acuity (with pinhole if worse than expected)
- intraocular pressure
- Seidel test (over bleb and anterior chamber paracentesis site, if present; see Ch. 32)
- check the peripheral iridectomy is patent
- note morphology of bleb
- depth of anterior chamber (especially lens- or iris-corneal touch)
- degree of inflammation
- presence of hyphaema
- presence of subconjunctival blood
- look for choroidal effusions (usually not present on day one).

Small leaks often settle down quickly with or without the use of a bandage contact lens (and a change in eyedrops to preservative-free forms). Discuss all findings with your senior if you are not confident of the requisite management.

Ongoing postoperative management is often complex, as failure of trabeculectomy is most likely in weeks 1–2. In the presence of marked inflammation of the conjunctiva forming the bleb, injection of further 5FU into the surrounding conjunctiva is not uncommon.

Squint surgery

JP Kersey

Introduction

Only a few years ago, squint surgery was one of the first operations learnt as a junior ophthalmologist, but more recently it has become a more subspecialised area. The techniques behind strabismus surgery are relatively simple and the real challenge lies in identifying which operation to perform.

Indications

The main indication for strabismus surgery is cosmesis, i.e. straightening the eyes; this is true in both adults and children. However, there are a small number of patients who derive a functional result from squint surgery (i.e. binocular single vision), for whom surgery is more than just a cosmetic operation. Another reason to operate is for the relief of diplopia in adults with late onset strabismus, usually from a nerve palsy or restrictive orbital disease, such as thyroid eye disease or following trauma.

It is important to identify why the procedure is being performed and the possible outcomes, and to explain this in detail to the patient, as they may have different expectations.

Prior to surgery, it is also paramount (usually through three sequential orthoptic measurements) to ensure that the squint is not still evolving. If changes in the squint measurements are noticed between clinic visits, it is not generally safe to proceed to surgery.

Basic principles

Squint surgery involves adjustments to the relative positions of the extraocular muscles on the globe, in order to align the visual axes. Individual muscles can be weakened or strengthened (in combination with other muscles) to achieve a satisfactory result. Either eye may be operated on to correct a squint, a fact that is often difficult for patients (and parents) to grasp. *Surgery is only performed after amblyopia has been treated and an appropriate refractive correction (if required) is in place.*

The commonest form of squint surgery is horizontal muscle surgery, which is performed for either esotropias (eye turning in) or exotropias (turning out). The procedure is usually performed to improve the patient's appearance and will not alter visual acuity, only rarely permitting the development of binocular single vision. The operation can actually induce diplopia if the child is unable to maintain suppression (of the deviating eye) following surgery.

Resection or recession?

A muscle is weakened by removing it from its insertion and moving it further back around the globe (*recession*), effectively lengthening it and so weakening its effect. Conversely, a strengthening procedure can be performed by removing a portion of the muscle (*resection*), thus shortening it, which increases its strength of action. If the eye is esotropic, then the medial rectus is recessed (put backwards) and/or the lateral rectus is resected (shortened).

There remains some debate about whether to operate on one eye or two in congenital cases. Some centres will routinely perform a bimedial recession for congenital esotropia, while other centres will routinely perform a unilateral recess/resect procedure. The degree of concomitance of the squint (i.e. the change in nature of the squint in different positions of gaze and the effect of spectacles on the squint) also affects this decision.

Selection and preassessment of patients

Squint surgery generally needs to be performed under general anaesthesia, as extraocular muscle manipulation is uncomfortable. Furthermore, excessive pulling on the muscles can activate the oculocardiac reflex, which can cause profound bradycardia (and even asystole). The patients must therefore be assessed for their fitness for a general anaesthetic, as well as their suitability for the specific operation.

Patients should have an up-to-date orthoptic assessment or documentation of a prism cover test in the nine positions of gaze. They should also have undergone a 'postoperative diplopia test', which involves using prisms to align the eyes as they would be after surgery, to ensure that the planned change in ocular position does not induce intractable diplopia.

If the patient has a significant refractive correction (usually hypermetropia in esotropia; see Ch. 6), this should be in use at the time of orthoptic assessment, as the measurements obtained may change considerably depending on the refractive state of the patient (occasionally abolishing a squint altogether, as in fully accommodative esotropia).

Consent

The following list should cover most postoperative eventualities:

- red eye
- discomfort
- need to use postoperative drops
- diplopia
- need to continue to wear spectacles postoperatively
- over-correction
- under-correction
- further surgery ($\approx$1:10)

- ocular perforation (rare)
- blindness (rare)
- general anaesthetic complications.

The procedure

The following description covers the commonly performed muscle recession procedure for a left congenital esotropia:

- The patient is anaesthetised using general anaesthesia and (usually) muscle relaxants.
- The eye is cleaned with povidone-iodine.
- A limbal conjunctival peritomy is performed between 8 and 10 o'clock (nasally).
- Superior (and often) inferior relaxing incisions are made radially towards the medial canthus.
- The flap is reflected and the muscle is identified.
- Tenon's fascia is dissected from the muscle.
- A squint hook is inserted along the sclera behind the muscle to hook it.
- A second squint hook is inserted from the opposite direction to ensure all of the muscle has been hooked.
- Remaining Tenon's fascia is removed from the muscle.
- Cautery is applied if needed.
- A 6/0 double-armed Vicryl suture is passed through the central portion of the muscle at the insertion.
- The suture is weaved thorough the muscle and locking sutures are placed through each edge of the muscle.
- The distance of the muscle from the limbus is measured.
- The muscle is removed from the insertion.
- The desired distance for reinsertion is then measured and marked.
- Sutures are placed through partial thickness scleral bites at the desired distance and then at the old insertion to form an anchored hangback (Fig. 51.1).
- Sutures are then tied at the old insertion.
- The conjunctiva is replaced to its original position and closed with 6/0 vicryl.
- Sub-Tenon's betamethasone and topical chloramphenicol can be used.
- The eye is then padded.

A resection is performed in a similar way except:

- After the Tenon's fascia is removed from the muscle, the amount to be resected is marked.

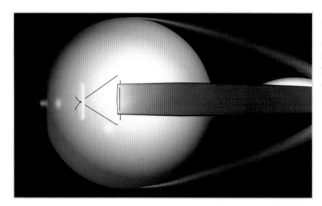

Fig. 51.1 Strabismus anchored hangback suture. Note the partial thickness scleral bites on either side of the new insertion.

- Sutures are placed just behind that point with double armed 6/0 vicryl, central and peripheral locking sutures.
- The muscle is cut anterior to the sutures and at the insertion.
- The spare muscle is discarded.
- The muscle is sutured to the insertion with partial thickness scleral bites.

Postoperative follow-up

- Day one: treat any discomfort and ensure there is no marked under- or over-correction.
- Week one: ensure the eye remains comfortable and there is no marked deviation. Ask about double vision.
- Month one: check the deviation and if possible measure it. Remind the patient things are still healing and there may be changes in the deviation over the next two months.
- Month three: ensure the deviation has remained satisfactory, and if not discuss with the patient whether any further surgery would be needed.

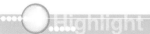Highlight

Squints: tips and pitfalls

- Always recess before resecting.
- Beware exotropias. They are not as common as esotropias and it is easy to do the wrong 'standard operation'.
- Fibrotic muscles in older patients can be secured on *adjustable sutures*, which can be altered after the patient has woken from the general anaesthetic to 'fine tune' the position of the eye.

52

Retinal detachment surgery

SV Raman

Introduction

New trainees in ophthalmology often perceive vitreoretinal surgery as a difficult speciality. This is partly due to the complexity of retinal tissue and its diseases, and partly due to the emphasis given to diseases of the anterior segment during the initial stages of training. Nevertheless, regular use of lenses and routine retinal examination will quickly allow the junior ophthalmologist to master techniques of examining the posterior segment and also to identify and understand its pathology.

For techniques of retinal examination, see Chapter 13 ('Indirect ophthalmoscopy') and Chapter 33 ('Retinal examination at the slitlamp'). This brief introduction to retinal surgery will help beginners in understanding the basics of some of the commoner vitreoretinal procedures.

Retinal detachment: pathophysiology

The process of retinal detachment is related to the presence of breaks in the neurosensory retina; a retinal break (hole or tear) is a full-thickness defect in this layer. Such breaks develop either due to inherent weakness of the retina, abnormal vitreoretinal adhesions or both. Horseshoe tears, which often lead to retinal detachment, occur during the process of posterior vitreous detachment. Atrophic round holes in the retina, which are also implicated in detachments, often develop in patients with 'lattice' retinal degeneration.

The posterior hyaloid, while separating from the retina during a posterior vitreous detachment, can tear a blood vessel or the retina, producing a vitreous haemorrhage or a retinal break (respectively), or both. Disruption of the sensory retina, as in a retinal break, also allows retinal pigment cells to gain access into the vitreous cavity. Thus, the presence of pigment cells in the vitreous (*Schaffer's sign*) warrants a thorough search for a retinal break.

A retinal break can progress to a retinal detachment when fluid from the vitreous gains access to the subretinal space and pushes the neurosensory retina forwards off the underlying retinal pigment epithelium (Fig. 52.1). In horseshoe tears, ongoing traction from the vitreous keeps the tear open, encouraging the ingress of subretinal fluid.

Principles of retinal reattachment surgery

- Close the retinal hole by approximating the neurosensory retina to the retinal pigment epithelium (RPE).

Common ophthalmic surgical procedures

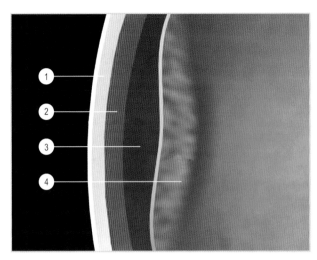

Fig. 52.1 Retinal detachment. Transverse section of the globe to illustrate a retinal detachment. Note that the sclera (1), choroid (2) and retinal pigment epithelium (3) remain in the normal anatomical position. The retina (4) becomes detached from the underlying retinal pigment epithelium.

- Drain or aspirate the subretinal fluid.
- Maintain closure of the retinal hole by creating a permanent adhesion between the RPE and the neurosensory retina (this can be achieved either by cryotherapy (freezing) or laser retinopexy).
- Relieve traction on the retinal break: an important factor that often keeps the retinal break from closing is ongoing internal traction from the vitreous, or scarring (proliferative vitreoretinopathy, PVR) on the surface of the retina.

The above steps can be achieved either by an external or an internal surgical approach.

External approach

Scleral buckling surgery (cryopexy & buckle with or without subretinal fluid drainage)

Suturing a solid silicone rubber band or silicone sponge on the surface of the sclera produces an internal indent, which approximates the RPE to the neurosensory retina. This, in effect, brings the RPE towards the retinal break, so obliterating the subretinal space, while at the same time reducing traction from the vitreous body on the retina. There are different sizes and types of silicone bands, and they may be used in a segment (*segmental buckle*) or around the entire globe (*encirclement*), depending on the type of detachment and associated pathology in the retina (Fig. 52.2).

The question of drainage of subretinal fluid is dependent on the amount of fluid present. Small amounts of fluid may be left alone for the RPE to pump out; however, larger amounts and fluid due to longstanding detachments will need to be drained in order for the retina to reattach. Carefully creating a track through the sclera, choroid and the RPE with a narrow bore needle allows drainage of subretinal fluid.

Once the retinal break is closed, a permanent adhesion needs to be created in order to prevent the break reopening with time. Applying a freezing treatment (cryopexy) across the sclera sets up a sterile inflammation in the choroid, RPE

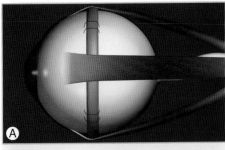

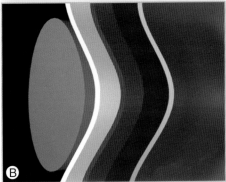

Fig. 52.2 Scleral buckle. A. The buckle is illustrated in blue and, in this example, encircles the globe. It is placed under the rectus muscles and is sutured to the sclera. **B.** Transverse section though an eye with a buckle. Note that the sclera, choroid and retinal pigment epithelium have been indented to lie against the detached retina, supporting it and relieving vitreous traction.

and the retina. This subsequently leads to chorioretinal scar formation, which firmly binds these structures around the area of the treated retinal tear or hole. Laser retinopexy achieves similar scar formation by inducing thermal damage.

DACE procedure

The acronym DACE stands for Drainage (subretinal fluid drainage), Air (injection of air or gas bubble into the vitreous cavity), Cryopexy and Explant (creating an internal indent by suturing a silicone band on the external surface of sclera). DACE works according to the four principles of retinal reattachment surgery described above. Drainage of subretinal fluid usually makes the eye soft and this induced hypotony can occasionally lead to choroidal haemorrhage. After drainage, air or gas is then injected to replace the lost volume and this may also be useful as a tamponade agent. Strictly speaking, DACE is not entirely an external approach, as gas is injected into the vitreous cavity.

Internal approach (pars plana vitrectomy (PPV); Fig. 52.3)

- The posterior segment of the eye is accessed surgically by making incisions in the sclera (sclerostomy). The pars plana is the site chosen, as this is relatively avascular; this site also avoids inadvertent trauma to the crystalline lens in front and the retina behind.

- A minimum of three sclerostomies are needed for the procedure; hence the name three-port pars plana vitrectomy.

- The first port sited is used for securing an infusion cannula into the vitreous cavity. Two other ports (superonasal and superotemporal) are fashioned for introducing the light source and vitrector. While performing vitrectomy

Common ophthalmic surgical procedures

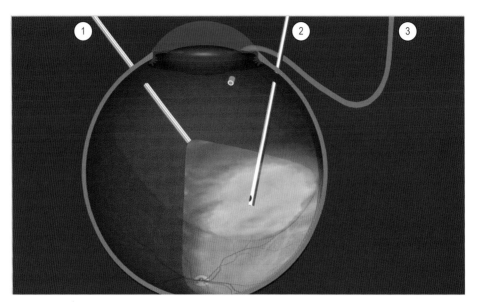

Fig. 52.3 Vitrectomy. There are three ports in the eye. Light pipe (1), cutter/vitrector (2) and irrigation (3). The bullous retinal detachment can be seen behind the vitrector.

surgery, fluid (BSS) is constantly infused into the vitreous cavity through the infusion cannula, so maintaining the structural integrity and shape of the globe. Following vitrectomy, an aspirating instrument is introduced into the vitreous cavity, and subretinal fluid is aspirated through the retinal break.

- Once the neurosensory retina is approximated against the RPE, laser (retinopexy) is applied around the retinal break(s) to create an adhesion between the two structures.

- It takes a few weeks for a firm scar to form. To prevent the retina from detaching while the scar matures, a gas bubble is injected into the vitreous cavity to keep the retina apposed to the RPE (internal tamponade). Air is usually not injected as this would be absorbed within a few days; the commonly used gases are SF_6 (sulphur hexafluoride) and C_2F_6 or C_3F_8 (perfluorocarbons).

- The gases take approximately 2 (SF_6) to 8 weeks (perfluorocarbons) to absorb completely. Patients are strictly advised not to undertake air travel while the gas bubble is still in the eye.

- In selected cases, the retina is further supported by suturing a buckle on the surface of the sclera (as in the external approaches described above). More complex retinal cases often require silicone oil as a tamponade agent to be placed in the vitreous cavity rather than gas. The oil does not dissipate and will need to be removed at some point in the future, but will of course provide support to the retina until such time.

Consent for vitreoretinal procedures

The following (non-exhaustive) list contains the most important issues to be covered when obtaining consent for vitreoretinal procedures:

- Blindness.
- Infection ($\approx$1:1000).
- Severe intraocular haemorrhage ($\approx$1:3000).
- Anatomical success rate for primary retinal detachment repair (i.e. retina reattached) varies between 80 and 95%. This is not the same as a return of normal vision, which depends to a large extent on the extent of a detachment (see below).
- Patients should be warned of the possibility of multiple further operations.
- Progression of visually significant cataract after vitrectomy occurs in nearly 50% of patients within a year, requiring a cataract extraction at a later date; a cataract will nearly always develop in a vitrectomised eye at some point in the future. As a result, some units are performing phacovitrectomy as a combined primary procedure in presbyopic patients.
- Patients should be warned of the need for gas bubble to be injected into their eye if they develop iatrogenic (entry site) retinal breaks (5–10%).
- Postoperative increased intraocular pressure may require medication.
- Diplopia (due to a buckle interfering with muscle movements) is also a possibility.

Further issues to be discussed prior to surgery

- Patients are often disappointed and alarmed if they are unable to see immediately after the eye dressing is removed. This may be misconstrued as a failed operation or a complication of surgery. Adequate counselling before surgery will allay some of the concerns and confusion after surgery.
- Visual recovery following vitreoretinal procedures is often not as dramatic as is generally the case after cataract surgery. The final visual acuity will depend on the status of macular function preoperatively. 'Macula-on' retinal detachments have a better prognosis than 'macula-off' detachments.
- The final visual acuity of macula-off retinal detachments cannot be predicted with certainty, but some patients can expect ongoing visual improvement with the passage of time. Repair of longstanding macula-off retinal detachments usually leads to patients regaining some peripheral vision, but central vision is nearly always permanently compromised.
- The presence of a gas bubble significantly interferes with vision; they are also responsible for producing strange entoptic images, often described by patients as bubbles, crescents, etc. Patients should be advised not to drive until the gas bubble has absorbed.
- Gas is often used to tamponade retinal breaks (see above). As gas floats on liquid, it may be necessary to adopt a particular posture in the postoperative

period in order to place the gas bubble against the responsible part of the retina. 'Face down' and 'left cheek to pillow' etc. are commonly found in surgeons' postoperative instructions and should be carried out for at least a few days. Specially designed pillows exist to help patients with posturing.

Medical postoperative care

Trainees in ophthalmology are not usually entrusted with seeing postoperative vitreoretinal patients alone by themselves. However, the following are usually noted on the first day:

- Visual acuity (usually poor, worse in a gas-filled eye due to induced hypermetropia).
- Degree of conjunctival inflammation.
- Anterior chamber inflammation.
- Crystalline lens for gas cataract, if gas had been injected into a phakic eye.
- Corneal endothelial debris. In face down posturing, debris accumulates on the endothelium due to the effects of gravity. This is often used as an indicator of patient compliance with posturing.
- Intraocular pressure.
- In a gas-filled eye, the amount of gas fill is noted. This is usually expressed as a percentage, e.g. 50% signifying approximately half the vitreous cavity being filled with gas, etc.
- The retina is checked for reattachment. The internal indent produced by the buckle and the position of the tear in relation to the internal indent are noted. The tear should be on the summit of the internal indent for the surgery to be optimally successful.

Postoperative management is an ongoing process and it usually takes a few weeks to months before it can be said with confidence that the retina is reattached.

53

Eyelid surgery

MJ Hawker

Introduction

Anatomical malposition of the eyelids can have serious consequences for the health of the cornea. Poor distribution of the tear film, irritation by eyelashes and exposure and drying of the cornea can all contribute to corneal scarring and perforation. Much of eyelid surgery (oculoplastic surgery) is aimed at restoring normal anatomical function of the eyelids to maintain a healthy cornea and good vision. In addition, the eyes are also very important cosmetically and there is always an element of cosmesis in the patient's and surgeon's thoughts. Lid surgery therefore needs to be performed well and is not an opportunity to just 'have a go'. Whilst there are many different indications for surgery of the eyelids, this chapter will concentrate on lid malpositions: specifically lower lid entropion, ectropion and ptosis of the upper lid.

Indications

Whilst indications for surgery will vary depending on the particular malposition, the main indications are:

- Discomfort to the patient as a result of lid malposition.
- Irritation and scarring of the ocular surface by eyelashes in entropion.
- Poor distribution of the tear film causing keratopathy (ectropion or entropion).
- Disturbance of vision by ptosis.
- Prior to cataract surgery (restoration of normal lid anatomy improves tear-film stability and may reduce the risk of endophthalmitis).
- Cosmesis.

Preassessment of patients

Nearly all lid surgery is performed under local anaesthesia. If the cause and associated morbidity of lid malposition has been adequately assessed prior to surgery, then the preparation of patients for surgery is generally straightforward. Whilst waiting for surgery, measures should be taken to minimise discomfort due to lid malposition. If lid malposition is adversely affecting the cornea, then a viscous tear substitute should be prescribed. If entropion is present, then surgical tape can be applied vertically underneath the eyelashes and stuck down to the cheek to evert the lid and prevent lash irritation.

Take a history to determine whether the patient is suitable for local anaesthesia as a day-case patient. Ask about any known allergies. If the patient is taking antiplatelet therapy (e.g. aspirin) or warfarin, make arrangements to stop the treatment prior to surgery if this can be done safely (a week before in the case of aspirin). Your unit should have a protocol for this situation. If ptosis surgery is planned, check for corneal sensation and Bell's phenomenon: if absent, the risk of corneal exposure following ptosis repair is greater (see Ch. 27).

Consent

Inform the patient of the expected course of events and any associated risks. In capable hands, the vast majority of procedures performed are successful.

- A degree of lid swelling and bruising is usual after surgery and should resolve by 2–3 weeks.
- If non-absorbable sutures are used these will have to be removed at the required time.
- The most common complications are related to excess swelling and bruising, especially if the patient is taking antiplatelet therapy or warfarin. In procedures where the septum is cut, there is a very small but definite risk of retrobulbar haemorrhage (≈1:40,000), which can permanently blind the patient unless treated quickly.
- Another common complication is related to under- or over-correction of the malposition, with the attendant need for further surgery.
- Depending on the procedure, a small scar may be visible. The risk of significant scarring is greater if the patient is known to have a tendency to hypertrophic scars or keloid.
- Rare complications include lid fistula and infection.

Postoperative care

- A pressure dressing is often applied for 24–48 hours to minimise swelling. Icepacks can be considered if required.
- Ensure that the patient has suitable oral analgesia to take if required.
- Many surgeons prescribe a short course of topical antibiotics (e.g. chloramphenicol ointment t.i.d.) for one week following surgery. Oral antibiotics are often prescribed if the orbital septum is cut (deliberately!) during surgery.
- Patients should generally be reviewed at one week to remove skin sutures if required and to check for over-correction or any other problems.

Specific procedures

Lower lid entropion repair

The most common cause of lower lid entropion is acquired involutional entropion in the elderly. Surgical repair aims to correct the anatomical factors that occur in ageing and contribute to entropion:

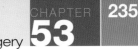

- increased horizontal lid laxity
- disinsertion of the inferior lid retractors
- overriding of the anterior lamella (orbicularis and skin) on the posterior lamella (tarsus and conjunctiva).

Surgical options include:

- Everting sutures:
  - These are quick to perform though provide only a temporary solution.
  - Three double-armed absorbable sutures (e.g. Vicryl) are placed through the conjunctiva near the fornix inferiorly to pass through the skin just below the lashes. Thus, when the sutures are tied, the lid everts.
- Wies procedure:
  - This is indicated when there is minimal horizontal lid laxity contributing to the entropion.
  - Using an eye guard, a full-thickness horizontal incision is made 4 mm below the lower lid margin (at the inferior border of the tarsus). Three double-armed everting sutures are placed through the conjunctiva and subconjunctival tissues (to include the inferior retractors) below the incision. The needle is passed to exit the skin 2 mm below the lash line. The skin is closed with 6/0 black silk and the everting sutures are then tied to form a minimal ectropion (which will correct when the anaesthetic wears off and orbicularis regains tone).
- Quickert procedure:
  - This is indicated for the correction of involutional entropion in the presence of horizontal lid laxity.
  - A 4 mm vertical incision (height of the tarsus) is made at the junction of the lateral one-third and medial two-thirds. A full thickness incision is then made 4 mm from the lid margin, across the width of the lower lid, ending medially below the punctum.
  - The final (vertical) incision removes an appropriate amount of the lid above this horizontal incision to address horizontal lid laxity.
  - 5/0 or 6/0 Vicryl is used for deep closure of the tarsus, ensuring good alignment to avoid a notch. The lid margin is closed with a grey line suture (anterior to the meibomian orifices) and a lash line suture. Everting sutures are placed as for a Wies procedure, and the skin is closed with interrupted sutures.
  - The lid margin sutures are removed after two weeks.
- Jones procedure:
  - This is indicated for involutional entropion without significant horizontal lid laxity.
  - A horizontal skin incision 4 mm below the lid margin is made.
  - Blunt dissection through orbicularis exposes the orbital septum, which is translucent and bulges due to the fat pad behind it. The septum is opened and the lower lid retractors, which lie just deep to the conjunctiva, are identified. They characteristically move on up- and down-gaze. Three to six 5/0 or 6/0 absorbable sutures are placed through the skin of the lower border of the wound, through the retractor and tarsus, emerging through the skin of the upper border of the wound. The skin is closed with interrupted absorbable sutures.

- Systemic broad-spectrum antibiotics are often given as a short course to avoid orbital infection (the septum has been opened).
- The procedure can be combined with a lateral tarsal (canthal) strip to address horizontal lid laxity. In this procedure, the lateral portion of the tarsus of the lower lid is resected and plicated to the lateral orbital rim.

Lower lid ectropion repair

The most common cause of lower lid ectropion is ageing (involutional). Other causes include mechanical, cicatricial (scarring) and paralytic (facial nerve palsy). In involutional ectropion the main contributors are:

- horizontal lid laxity
- reduced vertical skin tightness
- reduced orbicularis tone
- lid retractor weakness or dehiscence.

Surgical options include:

- Retropunctal cautery:
  - This is indicated for punctal ectropion and only addresses vertical components of the ectropion.
  - 2–3 rows of cautery burns are placed 4 mm below the punctum on the conjunctiva.
  - Scarring of the posterior lamella causes contraction and correction of the defect.
- Inverting sutures:
  - These address the vertical component of ectropion.
  - A diamond-shaped excision of conjunctiva and tarsus (dimensions ≈4 mm horizontal, ≈2 mm vertical) is performed with the apex of the diamond under the inferior punctum. Double-ended inverting absorbable sutures (e.g. 5/0 Vicryl) are placed through the inferior wound edge to pick up the lower lid retractors and to pass through the tarsus at the superior wound edge. The needle is then passed through the inferior wound edge to emerge on the skin side. The two arms are then tied to invert the lid.
- Lazy-T procedure:
  - This combines inverting sutures with lid shortening by wedge resection and therefore is indicated for ectropion with vertical and horizontal components.
  - The wedge resection is performed at the junction of the lateral one-third and medial two-thirds. Two vertical full-thickness cuts are made to extend 4 mm from the lid margin. The cuts are placed an appropriate distance apart to achieve the required amount of lid shortening. Two further cuts are made to form a pentagon of excised tissue.
  - The tarsus and lid margin are sutured as in Quickert's procedure.
  - The inverting sutures are placed as described above.
- Lateral tarsal (canthal) strip:
  - This is a lid-shortening procedure and only addresses horizontal components of ectropion.

- The lateral canthal tendon is exposed via a lateral incision over the orbital margin.

- The tendon is cut and a new tendon formed from tarsus. Skin and conjunctiva overlying the new tendon are removed and the tarsus is sutured to the orbital rim using a non-absorbable suture (e.g. Prolene).

- The superior and inferior lid margins are sutured to reform the lateral canthal angle, and orbicularis and skin are closed with an absorbable suture.

Ptosis repair

The majority of ptoses occur due to involutional deficiency of the levator aponeurosis. Further, less common causes include congenital levator dystrophy, neurogenic (Horner's syndrome or 3rd palsy) and myogenic (e.g. myasthenia gravis).

For involutional ptosis, surgical options include:

- Fasanella–Servat procedure:

  - This is indicated for mild ptosis (1–2 mm) where good levator function is present (see Ch. 27). Elevation of the lid is achieved through excision of upper tarsus adjacent tissues.

  - The upper lid is everted over a Desmarres retractor using a traction suture at the lid margin in the middle. Two haemostats are used to clamp the reflected lid including conjunctiva, upper tarsus and lower Muller's muscle.

  - One end of a double-armed suture is passed in and out of the tarsus, just adjacent to the clamps, to emerge through the skin at a lateral stab incision. The clamps are removed and the tissues excised along the marks of the clamps. The other arm of the suture is then passed along the opposite wound edge to achieve apposition and then emerges through the lateral stab incision to be tied.

- Aponeurosis surgery:

  - The levator aponeurosis lies deep to the orbital septum and superficial to Muller's muscle. Weakness or disinsertion of the aponeurosis due to ageing can be corrected by shortening the aponeurosis. Access to the aponeurosis is achieved via an anterior (skin) or posterior (conjunctiva) approach. Absorbable sutures are then placed to plicate the aponeurosis with the tarsus by an appropriate amount to raise the lid.

  - Postoperatively, oral broad-spectrum antibiotics are usually given as a short course to prevent orbital infection (the orbital septum is opened).

  - A detailed surgical description is beyond the scope of this text.

Corneal transplantation

ME Adams

Introduction

A corneal graft procedure replaces a diseased cornea with healthy donor tissue. It is one of the most frequently performed transplant operations.

The local transplantation service coordinates obtaining consent from relatives and the harvesting of donor corneas from cadavers, which must be achieved within 24 hours of death. Intermediate corneal storage at 4°C (5 to 7 days) and organ culture for longer-term storage (30 days) permits most cases to be scheduled electively.

Blood tests (hepatitis B and C, and HIV) and the analysis of previous medical and ocular history for potential donor suitability (and occasionally tissue typing) are completed. There is no age constraint to donors; however, endothelial cell counts must be in excess of 2300 cells/mm^2 in the United Kingdom.

Indications

The indications for a graft are optical (commonest), structural (e.g. in perforation of a corneal ulcer where corneal glueing is impossible) and cosmetic (disfigured eye). For optical (and therefore functional) indications, a graft can be considered when the cornea is the key limitation to achieving good vision. The optical integrity of the cornea is compromised and may necessitate a corneal graft in the conditions below (for example):

- keratoconus (commonest indication)
- Fuch's endothelial dystrophy and other dystrophies
- pseudophakic bullous keratopathy/aphakic bullous keratopathy
- interstitial keratitis
- herpetic keratitis
- corneal scars or ulcers.

Patient preparation

A healthy ocular surface and normal intraocular pressure are essential to optimise the chances of a successful graft; any pre-existing disease, especially glaucoma, must be treated prior to surgery.

Consent

Each surgeon may quote different complication rates. The following risks should be discussed with each patient prior to surgery:

- *Graft failure.* This may be defined as any irreversible change in the graft, preventing recovery of useful vision. Delayed clearing of the graft may occur (e.g. in diabetes), so a diagnosis of primary graft failure is usually not made until 2 weeks post-transplant.
- The leading cause of graft failure is endothelial cell loss following allograft rejection, which targets the donor corneal endothelium. Rejection is commonest in the first 3 months postoperatively, but may occur at any time during the life of the graft. Low-dose topical steroids are often used for the life of the graft to try and prevent rejection.
- Overall graft survival rates vary depending on the preoperative indication for the transplant. Patients with keratoconus and Fuch's dystrophy have a lower risk of graft rejection compared to other pathologies (e.g. herpetic disease).
- Risk factors which increase the risk of graft failure include the presence of anterior synechiae, deep stromal vascularisation, diabetes mellitus, perioperative ocular antihypertensive use, African-American recipient, larger recipient bed sizes and those patients receiving repeat grafts, for whom HLA-matched grafts and immunosuppression are often considered.
- *Astigmatism.* The patient must be warned of postoperative astigmatism and that refractive correction in the form of corrective lenses (contact lenses or spectacles) or even refractive surgery may be required. Full visual potential may not be achieved for up to 2 years postoperatively and will necessarily require the removal of corneal sutures during this time.
- *Recurrent disease.* Some dystrophies and infectious corneal conditions may recur and affect the success of the graft. In grafts performed for herpetic disease, oral aciclovir is often taken as prophylaxis for several years after the procedure.
- *Graft dehiscence.* The graft–host junction is vulnerable to even mild blunt trauma. Wound leaks postoperatively are often managed with a bandage contact lens but may occasionally necessitate resuturing in theatre.

The procedure

A corneal graft procedure may be broadly divided into full-thickness penetrating keratoplasty (PKP) or partial thickness lamellar keratoplasty.

A PKP replaces the full thickness of the central zone of the cornea and is the most frequently performed procedure. Lamellar keratoplasty transplants a disc of corneal stroma only and may be of any depth. A deep lamellar keratoplasty describes dissection down to the level of Descemet's membrane, leaving host endothelium in situ and so minimising rejection.

A further type of graft is the tectonic graft, which is the replacement of a section of structurally deficient cornea, e.g. in corneal perforation. It may also be of any depth.

Common ophthalmic surgical procedures

Most grafts will be done under a general anaesthetic; however, local anaesthesia is possible. Pilocarpine is usually administered to achieve miosis prior to surgery. Positioning of the patient is crucial to aligning the eye correctly, with the centre of the cornea vertically placed. This minimises any parallax errors during trephination procedures.

A brief outline of the stages in a PKP is given in the box below.

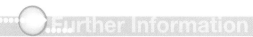 **Further Information**

Penetrating keratoplasty

1. *Select the graft size.* Trephines of different diameters are sized on host cornea; the ideal graft diameter is 7.5 mm. The larger the graft, the less the postoperative astigmatism, but the greater the risk of rejection (and vice versa).

2. *Excise donor cornea.* The donor corneoscleral 'button' is trephined to size, usually with the endothelial side up. Artificial anterior chambers are now becoming available that allow trephination to occur with the endothelial side down; this has theoretical benefits for reducing astigmatism.

3. *Excise host cornea.* Viscoelastic may be used in the anterior chamber to protect the lens. The host cornea is then carefully trephined—either manually or by motorised or vacuum methods. A partial thickness trephine and then diamond knife dissection may be performed to minimise the risks involved with a rapid decompression of the eye. The excised host tissue is always slightly smaller than the donor graft; this minimises postoperative leaks.

4. *Suture the donor cornea in place.* Monofilament nylon 10/0 is most often used. Four interrupted cardinal sutures establish symmetrical tissue placement and correct tension of the graft. Completion is either with interrupted sutures and/or a continuous running suture. Knots are buried in host tissue.

Postoperative management

The precise treatment regime may vary between different eye units and should be elucidated.

- Topical steroids are administered frequently to minimise allograft rejection. The frequency is reduced as seen to be appropriate at follow-up visits. Low-dose treatment may continue for years after a graft.

- A course of topical antibiotic (e.g. chloramphenicol) and a mydriatic may also be prescribed. All drops should be preservative free, at least until the graft has epithelialised. Prophylactic oral aciclovir 400 mg p.o. b.d. may be indicated in patients who received their transplant for herpetic disease.

- A bandage contact lens is sometimes used for comfort in the postoperative period.
- A meticulous slitlamp examination is essential at each postoperative follow-up.

Day one postoperatively

Watch for the following:

- Early graft failure, manifesting as profound cloudiness due to endothelial dysfunction. A degree of corneal oedema is normal after PKP.
- Loose sutures, or knots not buried.
- Wound leak—using the Seidel test (see Ch. 32).
- Iris prolapse.
- Flat anterior chamber.
- Raised IOP.

Subsequent postoperative visits

In particular, check for:

- Endothelial rejection—uveitis and keratoprecipitates at the graft–host interface, linear endothelial rejection line and stromal oedema.
- Epithelial rejection—linear epithelial rejection line and subepithelial infiltrates.
- Sutures—any broken or loose? Any evidence of adjacent neovascularisation or infection?
- Wound dehiscence.
- Glaucoma.
- Cystoid macular oedema.

In the event of epithelial rejection, intensive topical steroids will need to be commenced. Endothelial rejection is more serious and requires intensive topical treatment, often in conjunction with periocular or systemic steroid treatment (consult local policy).

Suture removal

Corneal topography allows the management of postoperative astigmatism with strategic choice of suture removal to adjust tension accordingly (see Ch. 4). Loose sutures will also need to be removed. Sutures are removed gradually after the graft–host interface has healed (usually after 3–6 months, check local policy). Sutures are usually cut with a needle and then carefully extracted with fine forceps from the host side of the cornea (pulling a cut suture through the donor side can occasionally lead to dehiscence of the graft–host junction or formation of a step). Following suture removal, cover with an increased dose of preservative-free topical steroid and antibiotic for a week.

55

Dacryocystorhinostomy (DCR)

ME Adams

Introduction

The aim of the procedure is to create a new passageway for tear drainage from the lacrimal sac directly into the nasal cavity, bypassing the obstructed nasolacrimal duct (NLD). This is achieved by removal of bone and the creation of a direct anastomosis between the lacrimal sac and nasal mucosa.

Indications

A DCR may be indicated in the following conditions:

- Epiphora with a blocked NLD. Syringing of the canaliculi must be performed in clinic prior to surgery to ensure patency of the drainage system for tears proximal to the lacrimal sac, confirming that the NLD is the site of blockage for tear drainage.
- Persistent mucocoele.
- Recurrent dacryocystitis.
- A DCR is also sometimes used to treat patients with functional block, i.e. epiphora when patent to syringing (but normal lid anatomy etc.). In this context, the success rate for the procedure is greatly reduced.

Patient preparation

The procedure is usually performed under a general anaesthetic (GA). When considering surgical treatment, the patient must be advised to weigh up the benefits of treating the symptoms of a watery eye with the operative and anaesthetic risks.

Blood loss can be significant, occasionally to a level which may threaten haemodynamic stability. Thus, a thorough clerking (with appropriate investigations) must be carried out to confirm fitness for surgery under GA. Drug history is vital. Unless medically inadvisable, patients on aspirin should probably be instructed to stop at least one week prior to surgery. Patients on anticoagulants, or those with clotting abnormalities, are probably not suitable without serious consideration.

Types of DCR

- Conventional DCR.
- Endoscopic DCR.
- Endolaser DCR.

As it is easily the most commonly performed procedure (and has the highest success rate), only conventional DCR is discussed below.

Consent

The published success rate of conventional DCR is ≥ 90%. Below is a list of potential complications that should be discussed prior to surgery:

- Perioperative haemorrhage.
- Postoperative haemorrhage.
    - mild, leading to periorbital bruising, small nose bleed or blood in tears
    - severe, may need hospital attendance, nasal packing and occasionally transfusion
- Scar.
- Infection.
- Failure to resolve symptoms < 10% (but ≈50% in functional block).
- Sump syndrome (rare): a stagnant pool of secretions, which collects in the old sac; requires redo surgery.
- CSF rhinorrhoea (rare) if the subarachnoid space is inadvertently entered.

The procedure

As a junior ophthalmologist, the DCR is not a great spectator sport, due to poor visibility and a small access port. If the effort is made, however, it provides an excellent demonstration of the anatomy.

Preparation

Asepsis and anaesthesia are assumed. A degree of hypotension, head-up posture and infiltration of a local anaesthetic (with adrenaline) at the site of skin incision will help to minimise bleeding. In addition, the nose is packed with ribbon gauze, soaked in cocaine, for vasoconstriction of the nasal mucosa. Xylometazoline nasal spray may also be used preoperatively.

Incision

This is carefully placed to avoid the angular vein and positioned on the flat of the nose to avoid subsequent bowstringing of the scar. The incision is usually ≈2 cm in length, starting just superior to the medial canthal tendon. Blunt dissection is used to traverse tissue planes, and the superficial medial canthal tendon is identified and cut.

Strip periosteum

This exposes the floor of the lacrimal fossa.

Osteotomy

This is the removal of sufficient bone to allow a successful DCR, generally about 2 cm × 2 cm. Extreme care is essential to avoid damage to the underlying nasal mucosa.

Create nasal flaps

These are to be later anastomosed to the lacrimal sac flaps.

Opening of lacrimal sac and creation of lacrimal flaps

A probe is passed through the canalicular system to tent up the lacrimal sac prior to incision. If asked to assist with this part of the procedure, advance the probe gently, with the lids under lateral traction, to avoid creating a false passage. Tubes may be used at this stage to try to ensure postoperative patency of the new system.

Anastomosis of nasal and lacrimal flaps

The flaps are opposed and sutured, posterior layers first. The anterior flaps can then be sutured to complete the anastomosis.

Closure

Skin closure varies widely, with some surgeons preferring to use non-absorbable sutures (e.g. silk or Prolene 6/0) while others use absorbable sutures (e.g. 7/0 Vicryl).

Follow-up

Prophylactic oral antibiotics are usually given (e.g. Augmentin 375 mg t.i.d. for one week). Topical application of corticosteroids (e.g. betamethasone) and antibiotics (e.g. chloramphenicol) may also be prescribed.

The patient should be reviewed prior to discharge from hospital. Attention should be paid to:

- Analgesia if required.
- Adequate haemostasis.
- Check the position of the tubes—ensure no ocular surface irritation.
- Ensure that the patient is aware of the need not to blow the nose forcibly (and to protect the anastomosis by occlusion of the nostril on the operated side, e.g. if they sneeze) for at least two weeks.

Follow-up at one week:

- Removal of skin sutures.
- Look for any signs of soft tissue infection.

Three month follow-up:

- Removal of tubes if required. After a brief check that the tubes are visible in the nose, cut the tubes at the medial canthus and ask the patient to 'blow your nose'; the tubes should come out of the nose. If they do not appear, an indirect ophthalmoscope and blunt forceps can be used to extract the tubes. If there is difficultly in identifying the tubes, topical nasal spray (e.g. phenylephrine) can aid nasal mucosa vasoconstriction to afford a better view.
- A nasal endoscope can prove to be very helpful in experienced hands.

56

Treatment of chalazia

R Sidebottom

Introduction

A chalazion or meibomian cyst is an inflammatory collection within the meibomian glands of the tarsal plates. It is not infectious in origin, though may follow an episode of internal hordeolum (meibomian stye).

Treatment

Conservative treatment involves lid hygiene and warm compresses to the lids; this may help to open the meibomian orifices and allow the cyst to drain. These measures are usually continued for at least four weeks before surgical intervention is planned. Many lesions will resolve in this time. For persisting lesions, surgery or steroid injections are indicated.

Surgery

This is a task which often falls to the junior ophthalmologist or nurse practitioner.

- Obtain consent from the patient. They should be told that local anaesthetic will be used, the procedure may cause local bleeding and a black eye, there is a small risk of infection and that it is likely that either other lesions may appear or that the chalazion may recur.

- Ensure that you examine and remember the size and location of the lesion very carefully initially, because after injection of anaesthetic and application of the clamp it is often a lot less obvious. A safer alternative is to mark the skin over the eyelid margin with a pen to ensure the correct area is incised.

- The area is anaesthetised with topical benoxinate (or similar) and 2% lidocaine with adrenaline (epinephrine) injection around the lesion, through the skin of the lid.

- The chalazion clamp is then applied with the flat surface to the skin and the ring encircling the lesion on the palpebral conjunctival side. The lid is then everted.

- Using a number 11 Bard Parker blade, the lesion is incised vertically through its conjunctival surface and then its contents removed using a small curette.

- The clamp is then removed. Chloramphenicol ointment (or similar) is then applied and the eye is padded for 2–4 hours. Antibiotic ointment should then be applied q.i.d. for five days.

- Future recurrences may be avoided by the use of warm lid compresses, as mentioned above.

Injection of corticosteroid

Some centres now perform injection of triamcinolone directly into the lesion. This is performed either through the skin or conjunctiva with prior topical anaesthesia.

Chalazion pitfalls

- Sebaceous gland carcinoma may be mistaken for a recurrent meibomian cyst. If suspicious, discuss the management of such lesions with your senior.

- Cysts near the canaliculi may be better treated with steroid injection or conservative management. Cysts medial to the puncta are not chalazia.

- Failure to drain lesions can be avoided by only attempting larger lesions until sufficient experience has been gained.

- Ocular perforation when performing the anaesthetic injection has been reported—care is therefore required!

57

Temporal artery biopsy

SN Madge

Introduction

Temporal arteritis (cranial or giant cell arteritis, GCA) is a relatively common systemic condition of unknown aetiology affecting medium and large arteries (specifically those that possess an internal elastic lamina) of elderly patients. In addition to its typical symptoms of headache, scalp tenderness, jaw claudication, fatigue, loss of weight and appetite, fevers and sweats, the most devastating complication is that of sudden and irreversible bilateral blindness due to ischaemic optic neuropathy (death due to GCA has also been reported).

A diagnosis of temporal arteritis usually condemns an elderly patient to a relatively long course of oral corticosteroid therapy, which, of course, is not without side-effects. A positive temporal artery biopsy provides definitive evidence of the disease's presence, thus justifying such treatment, which may be otherwise questioned in the face of subsequent complications such as osteoporosis, hypertension and diabetes. It should be remembered, however, that histological absence of the disease does not exclude the diagnosis.

Indications

It must first be established what the role of the ophthalmologist is in performing a temporal artery biopsy. Many biopsies are performed at the request of a consultant physician (generally patients without visual symptoms); in such situations, the surgeon often acts merely as a technician for the procedure and ongoing care remains the province of the referring physician. In patients with visual symptoms, in whom temporal arteritis is suspected, high-dose corticosteroids have usually already been commenced by an ophthalmologist.

Biopsies are performed to:

- Confirm the presence of the disease in a patient in whom the diagnosis is likely (e.g. classic symptoms with very high ESR, CRP, platelets).
- Establish the diagnosis where there is clinical doubt.

It must be emphasised that biopsies cannot exclude temporal arteritis, as skip lesions are common in histological specimens from patients with the disease. In the absence of confirmatory histology, the diagnosis is therefore a clinical one.

The superficial temporal artery is chosen due to its ease of accessibility. However, other arteries, such as the occipital arteries, may also be sampled if required.

Basic principles

Under local anaesthesia, a segment of artery is removed. Haemostasis is established and the wound closed. The biopsy is then examined by a pathologist. The longer the specimen provided, the greater the chance of a positive result— a specimen length of 3–4 cm is usually adequate.

Selection and preassessment of patients

- Patients must be able to tolerate a local anaesthetic and cooperate with surgery, which usually takes 15–30 minutes.
- Attention must be paid to any aspirin or warfarin use, which increases the risk of haemorrhage.
- If the patient is a known vasculopath, the possibility of stroke occurring as a result of surgery must be considered. In the presence of severe bilateral carotid disease, extracranial shunting of blood to the brain via the temporal arteries will be interrupted by injudicious biopsy.
- If a patient has been receiving corticosteroid therapy for some time, the value of the procedure is questionable. (A time window of two weeks—from starting treatment to biopsy—has been suggested by some as acceptable).

Consent

Patients should be warned of the risks of:

- bleeding (peroperatively and postoperatively)
- a scar, which is often concealed by the hairline
- the possible need for further biopsy if histology is negative
- stroke and death, if appropriate (see above).

It should be clearly explained to the patient that the biopsy is not a treatment for the condition, but merely a way of establishing the diagnosis.

The procedure

The following description is purely designed as a brief introduction to the operation for the new ophthalmologist.

- The site for the biopsy is selected on the basis of several factors, including evidence of localised disease and the ability to locate the artery in different areas. The area immediately above and in front of the ear ('danger' area) is usually avoided due to the presence of facial nerves in the area.
- The course of the vessel is marked on the skin. Occasionally, Doppler equipment is needed to map out the artery.

- Asepsis and anaesthesia are assumed.
- For the best cosmetic result, the exact incision line should be orientated to follow the skin tension lines.
- A superficial incision is made into the skin. The artery itself is always found in the superficial temporal fascia, which lies below the subdermal fatty layer.
- Once the correct plane is identified, the full length of the incision is opened and the underlying superficial temporal fascia (and artery) is exposed.
- The artery is identified and freed up through blunt dissection along its course. Superficial temporal veins are occasionally mistaken for the artery; however, these tend to run on, rather than in, the fascia.
- A single throw of a knot is tied around the proximal end of the artery and the patient is questioned about any unusual neurological symptoms that may develop (see possible extracranial shunting, above).
- This proximal knot is then tied fully, followed by further knot placement at the distal end of the artery. If any branches of the artery are present, these are also ligated.
- The artery is then cut free and carefully removed to avoid crush artefact.
- Wound closure is usually performed in two layers and a tight pressure dressing (for 24 hours) is often applied.

The postoperative period

If non-absorbable sutures are used, these are generally removed at 5–7 days. Follow-up (with histology) should also be arranged. In general, patients are discharged on high-dose corticosteroids pending histological results.

58

Refractive surgery

PA Baddeley

Introduction

Surgery for refractive error has become the most rapidly advancing field in ophthalmology of the past 20 years and has quickly become a speciality in its own right. Although not usually practised in the public sector, all eye care professionals require at least a rudimentary understanding of the speciality. They will undoubtedly be asked questions on the topic and may also be involved in treating the postoperative complications. It should also be remembered that it is now routine practice to offer patients a choice about their postoperative refraction after cataract surgery; thus, refractive surgery already forms an integral part of public sector ophthalmologists' workload.

This chapter covers only the fundamentals of this exciting new speciality, giving an overview of this rapidly expanding field. A thorough understanding of optics is assumed (see 'Basic clinical optics' section).

Background

All four types of refractive error (myopia, astigmatism, hypermetropia and presbyopia) can be treated with refractive surgery. However, the majority of surgery has been performed for myopia and astigmatism. Surgery for presbyopia, and to a lesser extent hypermetropia, is still considered more innovative if not experimental, and hence any long-term effects are less clearly understood.

The two main refractive elements of the eye are the cornea and the lens, hence refractive surgery is directed towards altering the refractive power of one (or both) of these elements.

The air–anterior cornea interface is the most powerful refracting surface in the visual system. Corneal refractive surgery works by altering the anterior corneal curvature, either directly using incisions or indirectly by altering the thickness of the stroma and hence the anterior curvature. By replacing the lens, the surgeon can alter both the anterior and posterior lens curvatures and the refractive index. This is used in clear lens extraction.

Excimer laser corneal refractive procedures

These procedures all use the excimer laser (excited dimer, 193 nm coherent monochromatic light). This very short wavelength ultraviolet beam is maximally absorbed by the corneal stroma, leading to vaporisation of tissue. The excimer laser is capable of vaporising layers of 0.25 μm at a time, whilst having minimal disruptive effect on surrounding tissues.

LASIK (laser in-situ keratomileusis)

Laser in-situ keratomileusis is currently the most commonly performed refractive procedure and is well established as a treatment for myopia up to −8 DS. First, a suction device fixes the globe. This enables a microkeratome to advance across the cornea, splitting the stroma into an anterior and posterior layer. The anterior portion is reflected but remains attached at one side via a hinge (Fig. 58.1). More recently, femtosecond excimer lasers are being used to cut the flap directly, obviating the need for a microkeratome (intra-LASIK).

The patient is asked to fixate on a central light to help centre the treatment area to the visual axis; however, computer tracking software allows toleration of some eye movement during the procedure. The laser ablates a calculated depth of stroma. This central reduction in corneal thickness flattens the cornea and has occasionally been used to treat up to −16 DS. By ablating the periphery of the central corneal zone, the central corneal curvature steepens, and hence the procedure can be used for the correction of hypermetropia up to +3 DS. Finally, the flap is replaced and a bandage contact lens is placed on the cornea.

Complications often relate to the flap and include:

- loss of the flap (with the anterior stroma)
- wrinkling of the flap
- epithelial in-growth at the flap interface
- deep lamellar keratitis, otherwise known as 'sands of the Sahara'.

Poor fixation initially caused decentration of the ablation area, but this has largely been overcome with computer tracking software.

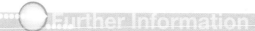

Further Information

Epi-LASIK

This is a very new technique that may combine the best of LASIK and PRK. A plastic blade is used to split the corneal epithelium at the level of the basement membrane, so producing a flap. This is retracted before the excimer is applied in the usual fashion.

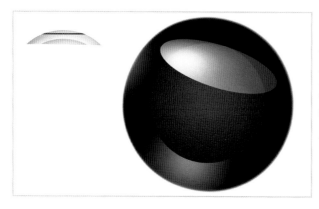

Fig. 58.1 Laser in-situ keratomileusis (LASIK). The cornea is shown in anterior (main) and side (insert) view. A flap is cut though the superficial stroma (red line) and reflected (as a flap) before the laser is applied to the underlying stroma.

LASEK (laser-assisted subepithelial keratectomy)

This procedure is similar to LASIK but uses an epithelial flap created after the application of 15–20% ethanol. Rather than the mid-stroma, as in LASIK, the anterior stroma is ablated and then the flap replaced (Fig. 58.2).

It is hypothesised that an epithelial flap decreases the production of extracellular matrix and collagen with a resultant decrease in postoperative haze. As the flap is more anterior than the LASIK flap, the most anterior stroma is ablated; hence, LASEK may be preferable in thinner corneas. Loss of the flap is also less important as the flap consists of epithelium only and will thus usually re-epithelialise within 48 hours.

LASEK has slower visual recovery compared to LASIK, as the epithelium may take up to 5 days to heal. Whether LASEK or LASIK produces better long-term refractive results has not yet been proven.

PRK (photorefractive keratectomy)

This procedure is the predecessor to LASIK and LASEK. It again uses the excimer laser, but instead of a flap, the epithelium is simply scraped away before applying the laser.

Afterwards the patient is fitted with a bandage contact lens, which remains for about 3 days until the epithelium is healed. By 2 weeks, subepithelial haze will be present which usually resolves by 6 months. This occasionally causes permanent glare and scarring.

Complications for all the above corneal excimer laser procedures

- Over- and under-correction.
- Infection.
- Glare disability and night vision disturbance.
- Myopic regression.
- Corneal scarring.
- Dry eyes.
- Reduced best-corrected visual acuity and contrast sensitivity.
- Inaccurate monitoring of IOP as central corneal thickness is decreased.
- Inaccurate IOL power calculations at subsequent cataract surgery (preoperative keratometry measurements should therefore be kept by the patient).

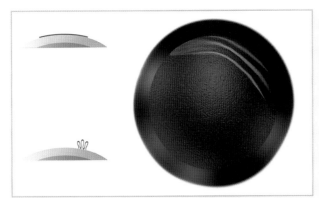

Fig. 58.2 Laser assisted subepithelial keratectomy (LASEK). After the application of ethanol, the epithelium (red line) is scraped aside and the underlying anterior stroma ablated.

Table 58.1 Orders of optical aberration important in wavefront analysis

Lower order aberrations	
2nd order	Myopia, hypermetropia, astigmatism
Higher order aberrations	
3rd order	Trefoil, coma
4th order	Tetrafoil, high-order astigmatism, spherical aberration
5th order	Pentafoil, trefoil, complex coma
6th order	Hexafoil, tetrafoil, complex astigmatism

The excimer laser and wavefront technology

Wavefront analysis is now often used to customise the excimer laser ablation pattern for each eye, which may help to achieve optimal postoperative uncorrected vision. Wavefront analysis involves the use of a laser beam reflected from a pinpoint on the patient's retina that is then received by a video sensor. From the perfect unaberrated eye, the reflected pattern should be a regular lattice of image points. If the reflected image is distorted, then computer analysis produces a wavefront consisting of many forms of optical aberration. Wavefront analysis can then be used to customise the excimer laser ablation pattern for each eye, so achieving optimal postoperative uncorrected vision.

Many orders of aberration exist; at present the aberrations that are analysed are from second order (i.e. myopia, hypermetropia and astigmatism) through to sixth order. Table 58.1 above lists some of these orders.

Other corneal refractive procedures

Radial keratotomy

This was the original refractive procedure for myopia, which flattened the anterior cornea by placing deep radial incisions whose origin, if extended, would meet at the visual axis. The centre of the visual axis is marked and a clear optical zone defined. The incisions are made with a diamond knife (to help unify depth) from the edge of the optical zone towards the limbus. The mid-peripheral cornea then bulges anteriorly whilst the central cornea flattens.

By modifying the number and depth of incisions the surgeon can alter the degree of refractive change produced. Age, sex, corneal thickness and preoperative curvature must be factored for when planning the procedure.

Radial keratotomy is well tolerated by most patients and is proven to be reliable and effective in low to moderate myopes (up to −6 DS). Its advantages include fast visual recovery and minimal postoperative pain. It is, however, not suitable for high myopes due to its unpredictability. It has now been superseded by PRK, LASIK and LASEK.

Limbal relaxing incisions

These incisions are used for the correction of astigmatism. These circumferential incisions are placed just anterior to the limbus, have a uniform depth of 0.6 mm and run for 6–12 mm length. The incision causes gaping and hence decreases the curvature in that meridian. The coupling phenomenon causes a steepening effect in the meridian at 90° to the incision. To ensure that the desired degree of effect is achieved, nomograms can be used which account for the size, number, and location of incisions, as well as the patient's age.

Intrastromal corneal rings

This involves the insertion of PMMA rings into the stroma of the mid-peripheral cornea, concentric with the limbus. They act as passive spacing elements, therefore shortening the arc length of the anterior corneal surface and hence flattening the central cornea.

Intraocular surgery for refractive error

Clear lens extraction and IOL insertion

Increasingly popular as an alternative to the above procedures is clear lens extraction with intraocular lens implantation. This procedure is identical to cataract surgery with the exception that the lens is not yet opaque. It carries identical risks to cataract surgery, most importantly infection, retinal detachment and postoperative macular oedema.

This procedure is likely to become increasingly popular as the technology of accommodative and pseudoaccommodative lenses improves. This would theoretically have three advantages: it would correct the refractive error, deal with the problem of presbyopia and remove the need for cataract surgery at a later date.

Intraocular contact lenses and phakic IOLs

There are now an increasing number of lenses available that may be placed within the eye to correct refractive error (e.g. iris clip lenses or phakic posterior chamber lenses). The technology is still evolving; however, if intraocular lens-induced cataract can be avoided, this approach holds great promise for the correction of myopia.

Section 6
Ophthalmic drugs

59

An introduction to ophthalmic drugs

JP Kersey

Introduction

Although the ocular pharmacopoeia is not as comprehensive as that encountered in other disciplines, many junior ophthalmologists will initially be very unfamiliar with the majority of the available ocular medications. This introduction to ocular pharmacology is just that; the different classes of available agents are briefly discussed in a pragmatic and introductory fashion. *It is strongly recommended that prior to prescribing any of the drugs mentioned in this chapter, the reader becomes familiarised with the relevant section in, for example, the British National Formulary.*

Examples of drugs in the different categories are given where appropriate. *These are not recommendations* and the reader is encouraged to elucidate local unit prescribing policies.

Mydriatics

These drops all dilate the pupil, but they do it in several different ways. Greater mydriatic power can be generated by combining drops from different groups. The anticholinergic group also have cycloplegic (accommodation paralysing) effects.

Sympathomimetics
- Adrenaline (epinephrine): this has poor penetration of the cornea and is now rarely used. It was used in the treatment of glaucoma some years ago (see below, in glaucoma medication).
- Phenylephrine (2.5–10%): an α_1-receptor agonist. It has good corneal penetration and is in routine use. The 10% preparation should be used judiciously due to the risk of potentially causing arrhythmias.

Anticholinergics
- Atropine.
- Homatropine.
- Cyclopentolate (1% for adults, 0.5% for use in young children and babies).
- Tropicamide.

These drops also act as cycloplegics (paralysing accommodation). They act to block postganglionic muscarinic acetylcholine receptors. Atropine can have

Ophthalmic drugs

significant systemic side-effects, including fitting and psychosis (see British National Formulary for exhaustive list), and must be used carefully in children. Its effects on mydriasis and cycloplegia may last for several weeks and therefore it should be used judiciously.

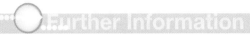

A comparison of the anticholinergic mydriatic drops

Tropicamide   Shortest

Cyclopentolate

Homatropine

Atropine   Longest lasting effects

Cocaine (4%)

Used in testing for a Horner's syndrome (see below). It acts by preventing the reuptake of noradrenaline (norepinephrine) at the neuron endplate, increasing its tissue availability and thus dilating the pupil.

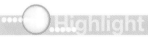

Mydriatics: tips and pitfalls

- Dilating drops can induce an increase in intraocular pressure (IOP), so IOP should be measured prior to dilatation.
- In patients with narrow angles, dilating the pupil can induce angle closure glaucoma. There is no danger, however, in patients with primary open angle glaucoma, a common misconception among non-ophthalmic physicians.
- Diabetic patients (particularly patients with long-standing disease) typically require both a sympathomimetic and an anticholinergic drop to achieve sufficient mydriasis for examination.

Miotics

These drugs are used to constrict the pupil. Initially used in glaucoma, they have also found a limited clinical use in reducing the size of pupils (e.g. if the edges of a pseudophakic lens are producing visual symptoms).

- Adrenergic antagonists.
- Opiates.
- Cholinergic drugs:
  - Pilocarpine (1–4%): see glaucoma medication below.
  - Miochol: often used intracamerally in cataract surgery to induce miosis.

Steroid eyedrops

These come in different strengths and as a result have greater or lesser side-effects. The main differences in their effects are due to differing penetration through the cornea.

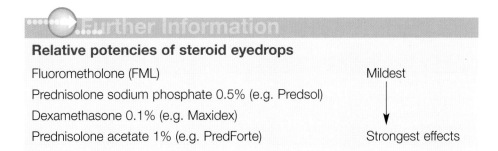

Further Information

Relative potencies of steroid eyedrops

Fluorometholone (FML)	Mildest
Prednisolone sodium phosphate 0.5% (e.g. Predsol)	
Dexamethasone 0.1% (e.g. Maxidex)	
Prednisolone acetate 1% (e.g. PredForte)	Strongest effects

Side-effects

- Around 20% of people on topical steroids show a rise in IOP after several weeks. If this is allowed to persist it can lead to a glaucomatous optic neuropathy.
- The majority of glaucoma patients (current or future) will show an IOP rise with steroids.
- A newer topical steroid, rimexolone, is said to be as efficacious as some of the stronger topical preparations without causing such severe IOP responses.
- Posterior subcapsular cataract with chronic use (also seen with systemic use).
- Inhibition of re-epithelialisation of cornea following injury.
- Mild immunosuppression—may be significant in the presence of contact lens wear.

Glaucoma medication

Drugs from different categories are often combined to produce an adequate reduction in intraocular pressure (IOP). As a result, some companies have produced combination drops in an attempt to increase patient compliance. Examples are given below.

β-blockers

- Timolol.
- Carteolol.
- Betaxolol.

This group of drugs remains a first-line treatment for glaucoma patients despite its long history. The main problems relate to the significant side-effect profile of

Ophthalmic drugs

β-blockers, which include cardiovascular effects (such as profound bradycardia), exacerbation of asthma, reduced exercise tolerance and occasional impotence in male patients. They work by reducing aqueous production and are typically administered twice daily. Some longer-acting preparations (once a day administration) are now available.

Adrenergic agonists

- Brimonidine.
- Apraclonidine.

Initially, topical adrenaline was used, but as it had significant side-effects (such as conjunctival injection and adenochrome deposits, as well as cystoid macular oedema) it fell from favour. More selective drugs are now available, in the form of α_2-agonists such as brimonidine. Although this drug does have a higher side-effect profile than some of the other medications (typically causes painful, red irritated eyes), it remains a useful second-line treatment. α_2-agonists are believed to work by decreasing aqueous production and increasing uveoscleral outflow. Apraclonidine is a shorter acting drug and is used mainly to prevent pressure spikes (and iris bleeding) following Nd:YAG laser procedures.

Carbonic anhydrase inhibitors

- Acetazolamide.
- Brinzolamide.
- Dorzolamide.

Inhibitors of carbonic anhydrase can be given in parenteral, oral or topical form. The systemically administered drug acetazolamide is used to reduce the IOP in emergencies such as angle closure glaucoma, or when patients are already on maximum topical therapy. These drugs act to reduce IOP by reducing aqueous production. They also constitute a useful second-line topical treatment.

These drugs have very similar molecular structures to sulphonamide antibiotics and should not be administered to patients with a documented allergy to such compounds. When systemically administered, side-effects are common, including tingling of the extremities, metallic taste in the mouth, diarrhoea, weakness, polyuria and potassium imbalance.

Prostaglandin analogues

- Latanoprost.
- Travoprost.
- Bimatoprost.

Prostaglandin analogues have been available for several years and have been shown to be extremely potent agents for lowering intraocular pressure. As a result, their arrival has led to a dramatic decline in the number of surgical drainage procedures that have needed to be performed. Although more expensive than topical β-blockers, they are now also considered first-line treatment for glaucoma.

They are believed to work by increasing the amount of uveoscleral outflow, possibly by remodelling of the extracellular matrix. There can be a delay in onset of action, with the peak antihypertensive effect often not being reached for several weeks. In addition, there is quite a long washout period for these drugs (again, several weeks). Approximately 15% of patients will not show a significant drop in IOP in response to a prostaglandin analogue.

Their side-effects are mainly mild: red eye from conjunctival hyperaemia, increased eyelash growth and increased iris pigmentation. Advantages of such drugs include their once daily application.

Miotics

- Pilocarpine (1%, 2% or 4%).

This drug has been long used in the treatment of primary open angle glaucoma to increase aqueous outflow but is often poorly tolerated in the longer term because of side-effects such as difficulty seeing in the dark, induced myopia and spasm. It is, however, still commonly used in the management of narrow angle glaucoma prior to Nd:YAG iridotomy. Constriction of the iris sphincter leads to the iris being pulled from the angle, so increasing aqueous drainage. It is also occasionally used in the treatment of pigment dispersion syndrome (and pigmentary glaucoma), by theoretically reducing chaffing of the posterior iris on the lens and zonules.

Pilocarpine has a marked side-effect profile including brow ache, impaired night vision and reduced visual field. A further drawback to its use is that it typically needs instilling four times a day.

Glaucoma eye-drop combinations

- Timolol and dorzolamide (twice daily administration).
- Latanoprost and timolol (once daily).
- Brimonidine and timolol (twice daily).

Hyperosmotic agents

- Glycerol is used to reduce the vitreous volume and so reduce the IOP in angle closure glaucoma and other causes of recalcitrant raised IOP. It is an osmotic diuretic, taken orally, and can often induce nausea.
- Mannitol is used to produce the same effect as glycerol. It is given intravenously as 1–2 g/kg over about 1 hour, usually as a 20% solution, and must be used with great care in the presence of a poor cardiac state. It will often induce a marked diuresis.

Ocular lubricants

Many conditions require the use of ocular lubricants, either temporarily to relieve acute ocular discomfort (e.g. corneal abrasion) or as long-term tear replacement in conditions such keratoconjunctivitis sicca.

Lubricants fall into three main categories, which show increasing viscosity. An increase in viscosity increases the length of action of the lubricant but also increases the length of time for which the vision is blurred after instillation. Manufacturers aiming to increase the first and reduce the second effect have developed gel-based lubricants, which make up the second category below.

Aqueous
- Hypromellose.
- Sodium Chloride (0.9%).

Gel
- Polyacrylic acid.
- Polyvinyl alcohol.
- Povidone.
- Carboxymethyl cellulose.
- Polyethylene glycol.
- Glycerine.

Ointments
- Liquid paraffin.
- Wool fat.

The aqueous drops blur vision for a few seconds, while the ointments can blur the vision for at least 30 minutes following instillation. This means that ointments are often best tolerated for overnight use, but are also used during the day in severe cases or when the vision in the affected eye is already poor. Ocular lubricants may have an impact on the ability of a patient to drive. In patients with tear deficiency, ocular surface mucin is often abnormal (often corneal filaments present) and the combination of a lubricant and a mucolytic (e.g. acetylcysteine) can be helpful.

Most drops are buffered to pH 7.7–7.8 and contain preservative. If the drops are required more than four times a day, then a preservative-free formulation should be used. As preservative-free formulations are often packaged in individual drop sachets, it may make financial sense for such products to be used in very infrequent-use patients, as bottles of preserved drops usually need to be discarded after 28 days.

Ophthalmic dyes

Rose Bengal
This is a corneal stain, which is used to identify devitalised tissue. It stains the edges of herpes simplex ulcers and also stains mucous filaments. It is quite uncomfortable to instil, so an initial drop of proxymetacaine is often used to reduce the patient's discomfort.

Fluorescein (typically 2%)

This dye is orange in colour and can be used for many purposes. When applied topically, it will stain corneal epithelial defects, the base of herpes simplex ulcers, demonstrate a leaking wound (Seidel test, see Ch. 32) and highlight the status of the tear film. It can also be injected intravenously (usually 10–20%) or taken orally (usually children) to allow a detailed study of the status of the retinal vasculature (see Chs 37 and 38).

Pharmacology tests

0.125% pilocarpine

The aim of this test is to identify denervation hypersensitivity in patients with a large pupil, e.g. Adie's pupil.

Method
Measure the sizes of both pupils. Pilocarpine 0.125% can be made by diluting 1% pilocarpine, 1 part to 7 parts sterile water. Instill one drop to both eyes.

Results
An Adie's pupil will constrict while the normal pupil will not.

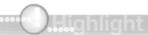

Adie's pupil: tips and pitfalls

- You need to note the pupils' sizes *before* instilling the drops, as well as after. The Adie's pupil is often larger than the other pupil before the drop is instilled so the pupils can end up the same size, which could be misinterpreted as a negative result.

- Denervation takes several weeks to develop so the test may be negative if the onset of symptoms is recent.

Horner's syndrome pharmacological testing

The aim is to first diagnose a Horner's syndrome pupil and then identify the affected neuron (i.e. pre- or post-ganglionic).

Drugs and results
Cocaine drops 4% prevent noradrenaline (norepinephrine) reuptake, so dilating a normal eye but not an eye with Horner's syndrome (interruption of the sympathetic nervous pathway leads to insignificant noradrenaline (norepinephrine) release).

Dilute (1:1000) adrenaline (epinephrine) will dilate a postganglionic Horner's syndrome pupil due to denervation hypersensitivity, but not a pre-ganglionic Horner's or a normal eye. Topical apraclonidine has recently been introduced into this field of investigation and works in the same way, relying on the principle of denervation hypersensitivity.

Ophthalmic drugs

The eye can be retested 48 hours later with 1% hydroxyamphetamine, which causes release of noradrenaline (norepinephrine) at the nerve terminal, so dilating a pre-ganglionic Horner's and normal eyes, but not a post-ganglionic Horner's.

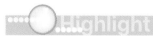

Horner's tests: tips and pitfalls

- The eye needs to recover from the effect of the cocaine before a second test can be performed (two days).
- Hypersensitivity takes time to develop, see above (Adie's pupil).
- If the results do not ring true, an MRI scan will often provide a definitive result.

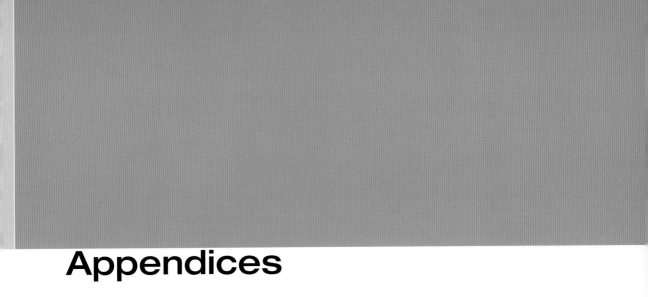

Appendices

An introduction to ophthalmic notes

SN Madge

Introduction

To a new ophthalmologist, ophthalmic notes are often indecipherable; orthoptic notes often remain as such until very late in one's training! Although there are many variations around the world, this section will provide a brief insight into some of the ways that you might find ophthalmic notes documented.

Please refer to the relevant chapters for more information, if required.

General remarks

With the exception of confrontational visual field examinations, notes concerning the patient's right eye are written on the left side of the page, whereas notes about the patient's left eye are to be found on the right (i.e. documentation as if you are looking at the patient in the notes). If there is any doubt, banish it by marking each side of the notes 'R' or 'L'.

For all ophthalmic notes, it is important to write clearly, legibly and always sign and date your entries. Particularly as a trainee, who may not be spending a long time within a particular department, it is helpful to print your name under your signature, along with a contact number. Particularly for orthoptic diagrams, check your local unit protocol, as there are many variations on the theme.

Notation and standard abbreviations

- Hx: history (sometimes HPC—history of presenting complaint). This section may include other abbreviations, which are often to be found in general medical and surgical notes, including:
  - PMHx or PMH: previous medical history.
  - POHx: previous ocular history.
  - DHx: drug Hx.
  - NKDA: no known drug allergies.
  - FHx: family history.
  - SHx: social history, including smoking.

Appendices

- O/E: on examination.
  - OD: right eye.
  - OS: left eye.
  - OU: both eyes together.
- *Visual acuity* (VA) (Snellen fraction, e.g. 6/6, 3/3, or logMAR score, e.g. 0.3). It should be stated whether the measurement is made with the use of spectacles ('aided') or not ('unaided'), and with or without a pinhole. Other abbreviations include:
  - NIPH: no improvement with a pinhole.
  - BCVA: best corrected visual acuity (i.e. with *contemporary* refractive correction in place).
  - BVA: binocular visual acuity.
  - 'Near' or NVA: near visual acuity (measured with the British N system or the Jaeger system).
- *Pupils:* L. RAPD means a 'left relative afferent pupillary defect' ('°RAPD' means no RAPD). PERLA is an abbreviation not usually used by ophthalmologists, but means 'pupils equal and reactive to light and accommodation'.
- *Visual fields* (VF), when documented, are recorded as if seen from the patient's perspective, e.g. a right superior homonymous quadrantanopia is documented as shown in Figure A1.1, with the blacked-out area representing the scotoma on the right side of space. It is useful to document the stimulus used, e.g. a red pin (or a flash-light if vision is markedly impaired).
- *Cornea:* variations abound, but many have adopted the recommendations of Waring & Laibson (1977). The cornea is usually depicted as a circle in the notes (≈35 mm in diameter), on which is drawn pathology. Numbers on corneal diagrams usually represent the dimensions of pathology in millimetres, as measured with the slitlamp. Corneal thinning is best documented by drawing a cross-section of the cornea, often accompanied by an estimate of

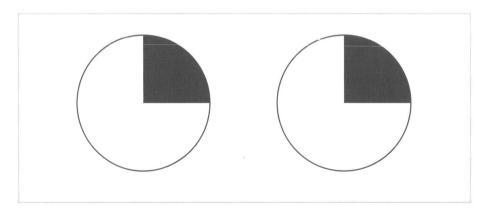

Fig. A1.1 Documentation of a right superior homonymous quadrantanopia, with the patient's right eye being documented on the right side of the notes.

thinning as a percentage. The colour scheme recommended by Waring & Laibson is as follows:

- Blue: oedema (lines = Descemet's folds, bubbles = epithelial oedema).

- Brown: pigment or iris.

- Green: scar or corneal degeneration, also for sutures or contact lens.

- Red: blood and vessels (dashed lines indicate ghost vessels).

- Green: fluorescein staining, also used for lens and vitreous.

- Orange: infiltrate, hypopyon, keratic precipitates.

- *Iris:* transillumination defects and peripheral iridotomies are simply depicted as holes in a coronal picture of the iris.

- *Intraocular pressure* (IOP): it is important to document the way that IOP is measured, as some techniques are more accurate than others. The use of the letter 'A' (see below) is usually taken to mean an IOP measured by an applanation technique (e.g. Goldmann or Perkins), whereas 'T' does not specify the method involved, simply meaning tonometry.

A	T
12 14	12 14

- *Anterior chamber* (AC): a normal AC is often abbreviated as 'd & q' or 'deep and quiet'. Shallow ACs (as in narrow angle glaucoma) should be mentioned clearly in full. 'Quiet' implies no cells or flare in the anterior chamber, as one might find in an inflammatory condition such as iritis. Cells and flare are often documented by the notations −/+, +/−, ++++/−, +/+, +/++++, etc., with the first symbol ('+' or '−') often referring to cells and the second referring to flare in the AC. As with any (subjective) method of recording clinical signs, the inter- and intra-observer variability is known to be less than optimal.

- Cells should be graded by counting the number of visible cells in an oblique slit beam at full intensity, high magnification, 3 mm long and 1 mm width. Common notations are:
  'Occ. cell': occasional cell seen
  +   : 5–10 cells
  ++   : 10–20 cells
  +++   : 20–50 cells
  ++++ : >50 cells but no hypopyon
  Hypopyon.

- Flare is graded in a more qualitative way:
  +   : just detectable
  ++   : moderate, iris details clear
  +++   : iris details hazy
  ++++ : fibrin present in the AC (often simply written as 'fibrin' rather than '++++').

- *Lens and cataract:* lenses are often drawn in two dimensions (coronal plane and sagittal plane), with the location of the cataract marked in by shading. The following abbreviations are commonly used:

- NS: nuclear sclerosis.

- 'Cort.': cortical cataract.

Appendices

- PSCO: posterior subcapsular opacity.
- ASCO: anterior subcapsular opacity (uncommon).
- LO: simply lens opacity.
- PCO: posterior capsular opacity (seen in pseudophakes).

- *Vitreous:* the commonest abbreviation found is probably PVD, which means 'posterior vitreous detachment'. Other abbreviations include:
  - TD: tobacco dust (often found with retinal tears).
  - AH: asteroid hyalosis.

- *Retina:* the retina is often drawn schematically in the notes as a circle containing the optic disc and the major vascular arcades; pathology is then marked on it as required. Some departments may still use retinal detachment charts for documenting peripheral retinal pathology in detachment cases. On retinal diagrams, retina is usually shaded blue if detached and red if attached, exudates are marked in yellow, retinal pigment in black and vitreous opacities in green (Fig. A1.2).

- *Eye movements:* these are documented in many different ways, but most departments' orthoptists use a consistent scheme, particularly for their abbreviations, which are legion. Some abbreviations are listed below:
  - CT: 'cover test' result, usually with results for near (e.g. $\frac{1}{3}$ m) and distance (e.g. 6 m).
  - E usually represents esophoria (e.g. 'R. E', right esophoria), and ET an esotropia. E(T) is an intermittent esotropia.
  - Similar notation exists for exodeviations, e.g. X, XT and X(T) for exophoria, exotropia and intermittent exotropia, respectively.
  - HT and HYPO mean hypertropia and hypotropia, respectively.
  - PCT denotes a 'prism cover test' result. As such, it will then be followed by some measurements in prism dioptres (Δ), which will be BI (prism 'base-in'), BO (base-out), BU (base-up) or BD (base-down), usually for distance and near. These are often measured in the nine positions of gaze.
  - An example of the method of documentation of eye movements popularised by Vivian & Morris (1993) is shown in Figure A1.3. This provides the results of prism cover tests (nine positions of gaze) and the ocular movements on the same

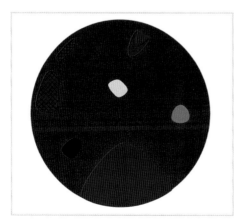

Fig. A1.2 Example of a retinal diagram (optic disc and vessels are often also marked for orientation purposes). The retina is shown here shaded blue if detached and red if attached, exudates are shown in yellow, retinal pigment in black and vitreous opacities in green. In addition, retinal thinning is shown as red hatchings outlined in blue, with lattice degeneration being shown as blue hatchings.

diagram. Versions are scored from −4 to +4, with 0 being normal, and are marked on the diagram in the nine diagnostic positions of gaze. In a normal horizontal version, no sclera should be visible at the canthus in the direction of movement (scores 0). If sclera is just visible, this is scored as −1; if there is an inability to move the eye more than half way into the field of action of the muscle concerned, this scores −2; less than a quarter of the distance scores −3; and an inability to move from the midline scores −4. As mentioned above, the patient's right eye is documented on the left side of the page (as if you were examining the patient).

An example of this system in action is shown in Figure A1.4, in the case of a right 4th nerve palsy, with secondary overaction of the right inferior oblique and left inferior rectus.

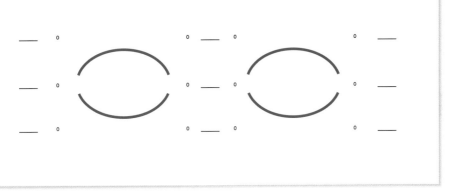

Fig. A1.3 The Vivian & Morris (1993) scheme for documentation of eye movements. '—' represents the location for documenting the PCT results (in prism dioptres) for the nine positions of gaze; '°' represents the location of the version results. On the diagram can be added curved arrows, representing updrifts and downdrifts, sloping vertical lines representing 'A' and 'V' alphabet patterns, and hashed areas which symbolise areas of restricted ocular movement.

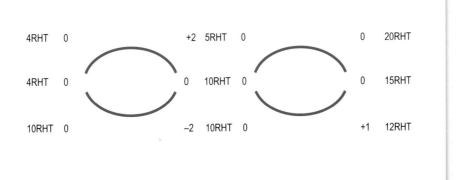

Fig. A1.4 An example of documentation of a right 4th nerve palsy, with secondary overaction of the right inferior oblique and left inferior rectus. The right hypertropia (RHT) seen in the primary position gets worse in laevoversion, due to right inferior oblique overaction (upgaze) and left inferior rectus overaction (downgaze).

Appendices

- *Ptosis measurements:* as well as a brief sketch of the contour of the lids, the following abbreviations are often found in notes. Measurements pertaining to the right eye are often to be found to the left side of the abbreviation, those for the left eye are to be found on the right.

  - PA: palpebral aperture (followed by the measurement in mm).

  - MRD: margin-reflex distance.

  - SC: skin crease.

  - LF: levator function.

Other lid abnormalities are usually described in full, or a brief diagram aids documentation.

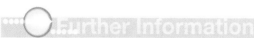

Further Information

Suggested further reading

- Waring GO, Laibson PR. A systematic method of drawing corneal pathologic conditions. Arch Ophthalmol 1977; 95(9): 1540–2.

- Vivian AJ, Morris RJ. Diagrammatic representation of strabismus. Eye 1993; 7: 565–71.

- Kanski JJ. Clinical Ophthalmology. 5th edn. Oxford: Butterworth Heinemann; 2004.

Visual requirements for driving and the registration of partial sight or blindness (United Kingdom)

MJ Hawker

Visual requirements for driving

The Driver and Vehicle Licensing Agency (DVLA) requires different minimum levels of visual function for Group 1 (ordinary car licence) and Group 2 (large goods vehicle, passenger carrying vehicle, medium goods or minibus) license holders. The reader should check its website for full details which may be subject to change (www.dvla.gov.uk). A summary of the major current visual requirements is given here.

The law states that:

'A licence holder or applicant is suffering a prescribed disability if unable to meet the eyesight requirements, i.e. to read in good light (with the aid of glasses or contact lenses if worn) a registration mark fixed to a motor vehicle and containing letters and figures 79 millimetres high and 57 millimetres wide (i.e. pre 1.9.2001 font) at a distance of 20.5 metres, or at a distance of 20 metres where the characters are 50 millimetres wide (i.e. post 1.9.2001 font).'

If unable to meet this standard, the driver must not drive and the licence must be refused or revoked.

Group 1 Entitlement (to hold a licence)

- The patient must be able to meet the above requirements (binocularly).
- If cataract is present, then glare caused by bright sunlight might prevent the patient meeting these requirements.
- If the patient completely loses vision in one eye, they must inform the DVLA. They may return to driving after an undefined period of adjustment to their monocular situation but only if they can meet the legal requirements for vision and the visual field is full in the good eye.
- Visual field status for driving is assessed using a binocular Estermann visual field test (target equivalent to Goldman III4e). The minimum field required is

at least 120° on the horizontal scale, with no significant defect within 20° of fixation above or below the horizontal meridian. Homonymous or bitemporal defects, which approach the central field (whether hemianopic or quadrantanopic), are not accepted as safe for driving.

- Acceptable central defects (within central 20°) are defined as scattered single missed points, or a single cluster of up to three contiguous missed points.

- Unacceptable central defects include a cluster of four or more contiguous missed points, one single cluster of three contiguous missed points if accompanied by additional single missed points, or any central loss that is an extension of hemianopia or quadrantanopia.

- If diplopia is diagnosed (whatever the cause), the patient must cease driving. Driving may be resumed after a period of adjustment if the symptoms are controlled with patching or prismatic correction.

Group 2 Entitlement

- Minimum uncorrected visual acuity of at least 3/60 in each eye.

- With correction, the better eye must achieve a minimum of 6/9 and the worse eye a minimum of 6/12.

- Outdoor acuity (which may unmask the effects of glare from cataract) must achieve the minimum legal requirement stated above.

- The group 2 license must be revoked if loss of vision in one eye occurs.

- Normal binocular field of vision is required.

- If diplopia occurs and symptoms cannot be controlled with prismatic correction, the license must be revoked (patching is not acceptable).

Certificate of Visual Impairment (2003)

In November 2003, the Department of Health introduced the new 'Certificate of Visual Impairment 2003' (CVI) to replace the old BD8 form. In order to reduce referral delays, two additional standard referral letters were produced: the Letter of Vision Impairment (LVI) for high street optometrists to give to people to self-refer, and the Referral of Vision Impaired Patient (RVI) for use within Hospital Eye Services.

The CVI is used to formally register a patient as 'Severely Sight Impaired' (blind), or 'Sight Impaired' (partially sighted). Registration is voluntary and enables access to various benefits in addition to triggering a referral for social care assessment. The form records the patient's personal details, visual acuity and visual field, and the diagnosis causing visual dysfunction. The form can only be signed by a consultant ophthalmologist, who (under the new consultant contract) will no longer be able to attract a fee for this service (unlike BD8). With the patient's consent, copies of the form are sent to the Local Authority, the patient's GP, epidemiological data collection, and copies are retained by the patient and in the hospital notes.

Severely sight impaired (blind)

The National Assistance Act (1948) states that a person can be certified as blind if they are 'so blind as to be unable to perform any work for which eye sight is essential' (National Assistance Act Section 64(1)). Note that it is the ability to perform any work, not just the patient's normal job, which is tested. Patients should be classified according to the following criteria:

- Patients who are below 3/60 (Snellen acuity):
  - Most patients who have visual acuity below 3/60 should be certified blind.
  - Patients who have visual acuity of 1/18 (slightly better than 3/60) should not be certified blind unless they also have considerable restriction of visual field.
- Patients who are better than 3/60, but below 6/60 Snellen:
  - Patients with a very contracted field of vision should be certified blind.
  - Patients who have had a visual defect for a long time, and who do not have a very contracted field of vision should not be certified blind (e.g. congenital nystagmus, albinism).
- Patients who are 6/60 or above:
  - Patients with a very contracted field of vision (especially in the inferior field) should be certified as blind.
  - Patients with homonymous or bitemporal hemianopia who still have central visual acuity of 6/18 or better should not be certified blind.

Sight impaired (partially sighted)

Patients are considered for sight impaired registration if they have a visual acuity of:

- 3/60 to 6/60 with full field.
- Up to 6/24 with moderate contraction of the field, opacities in the media or aphakia.
- 6/18 or better if they have a cross visual field defect (e.g. hemianopia, marked contraction of the visual field in glaucoma).

Glossary

A

Accommodation: the process by which a change in lens position and shape effects an increase in the refractive power of an eye, so allowing near vision.

Add: an additional positive (convex) lens added to a distance prescription (usually bilaterally) to allow near vision.

Adie's pupil: a clinical condition where a pupil is typically larger than the contralateral pupil and exhibits light-near dissociation, vermiform movements of the iris and hypersensitivity to pilocarpine. It is thought to represent denervation of nerves from the ciliary ganglion.

Against-the-rule: astigmatism of the form *plus* cylinder with an axis at 180 degrees, or *minus* cylinder with an axis at 090 degrees (c.f. *with-the-rule*).

Amblyopia: a (typically unilateral) failure of visual development, which is not the result of any clinically demonstrable abnormality of the visual system.

Ametropia: a condition where light is not focused onto the retina by the relaxed eye (e.g. myopia or hypermetropia).

Aniseikonia: a disparity in retinal image size between the two eyes, often as a result of differing refractive states (*anisometropia*) in the two eyes.

Anisocoria: a difference in pupil size between the two eyes.

Anisometropia: a difference in the refractive corrections between the two eyes (often only significant at greater than around 2 D).

Aphakia: an absence of the normal crystalline lens of the eye (usually surgical).

Astigmatism: a difference in refractive power in different meridia (see Ch. 3).

Axis: a method of defining the direction of action of an astigmatic lens (see Ch. 3).

B

Bell's phenomenon: the spontaneous elevation of the globe seen on closure of the eyelids.

Bifocal: a spectacle lens incorporating a distance vision segment and a near vision segment (the *add*).

Binocular single vision (BSV): the ability to use both eyes simultaneously, with each eye contributing to a single visual perception. Worth classified BSV into three stages: simultaneous perception, fusion and stereopsis.

Bleb: a surgically created subconjunctival space that allows drainage of aqueous humour from the eye (usually via a trabeculectomy).

Blebitis: an infection of a bleb.

Blepharophimosis syndrome: an autosomal dominantly inherited condition comprising ptosis, poor levator function, epicanthus inversus, telecanthus and short palpebral apertures.

C

Capsulorhexis: the surgical opening in the anterior lens capsule to allow modern cataract surgery.

Chemosis: subconjunctival fluid found usually as a result of inflammation (common in allergic disorders).

Commotio retinae: physical damage (usually by blunt injury) to the neuroretina causing cloudy swelling of the tissue.

Concomitant: a strabismus (squint) where the angle of deviation remains the same regardless of the direction of gaze (c.f. *incomitant*).

Coupling phenomenon: the principle that surgically induced changes in the cornea (e.g. limbal relaxing incisions or compression sutures) may change the power and axis of astigmatism but have no effect on the overall spherical equivalence of the cornea.

Critical angle: the angle above which total internal reflection of light occurs for a particular interface between two media of different refractive indices (e.g. cornea and air).

Crowding effect: the phenomenon that it is easier to read a single letter on a visual acuity chart than a cluster of letters (much more marked in amblyopes).

Cycloplegia: paralysis of the ciliary muscles leading to an absence of accommodation.

Cylinder: a type of lens which has no refractive power in one axis, but has a refractive power at 090 degrees to this axis (c.f. spherical and toric lenses).

D

D: abbreviation for dioptre.

DC: abbreviation for a dioptre of cylindrical lens correction.

DS: abbreviation for a dioptre of spherical lens correction.

Deutan: referring to the cones that are maximally 'green' sensitive in their spectral composition.

Dextroversion: the binocular movements of the eyes to the right.

Dioptre: the international unit for the vergence (focusing) power of lenses. A lens of 1 D strength will focus incident parallel light to a point at 1 m from the lens.

Dissociation: the process of functionally separating the eyes for the purposes of examination (e.g. Hess test, red–green goggles).

Ductions: uniocular movements of the eyes (c.f. versions).

Dystopia: an abnormal position of the globe per se (as opposed to the visual axis in a heterotropia (tropia)).

E

Emmetropia: the refractive condition of a relaxed eye that focuses parallel light on to the retina.

Enophthalmos: a condition where the eye is abnormally recessed within the orbit. It must be distinguished (e.g. by exophthalmometry) from pseudoenophthalmos, where the eye simply appears to be in such a position.

Esophoria: a condition where the visual axes are aligned during binocular viewing, but which become convergent on dissociation.

Esotropia: a condition in which one eye deviates nasally while both eyes are open.

Exophthalmos: this term has been used rather loosely to mean proptosis, but has also been used to denote proptosis in the setting of thyroid eye disease.

Exophoria: a condition where the visual axes are aligned during binocular viewing, but which become divergent on dissociation.

Exotropia: a condition in which one eye deviates temporally while both eyes are open.

F

Far point: the position of an object such that its image falls on the retina of the relaxed eye (i.e. with no accommodation).

Focal length: the reciprocal of the dioptric power of a lens, which is the distance from the lens that incident parallel light would be brought to a point focus (see Dioptre).

Fresnel prism: a plastic sheet of tiny parallel prisms of identical refracting angle, which function as a single large prism. These are often stuck on to the surface of spectacles to provide relief from diplopia.

Fusion: the perception of an object by each eye to form a unified single image of the object (fusion may be central or peripheral).

H

Heterochromia: a difference in colour of the iris between the two eyes.

Heterotropia (often abbreviated to tropia): the deviation of the visual axis of either eye (in any direction) while both eyes are open.

Hypermetropia, hyperopia: the condition where the relaxed eye is of insufficient power to focus parallel light on to the retina. Convex (*plus*) correcting lenses are required.

Hyphaema: the presence of blood in the anterior chamber (usually layered inferiorly, macrohyphaema).

Hypoglobus: a relative depression of the entire globe (not the visual axis as in hypotropia) compared to the other eye.

I

Incomitant: a strabismus (squint) where the angle of deviation changes depending on the direction of gaze, accommodation or which eye is fixing (c.f. *concomitant*).

Interpupillary distance: the horizontal distance between the centres of the pupils.

IOL: intraocular lens implant.

IPD: see *interpupillary distance*.

Iridodialysis: a separation of the root of the iris from the angle of the anterior chamber of the eye (seen in blunt trauma).

Iridodonesis: the spontaneous wobbling of the iris seen in cases of weak lens zonules or iridodialysis.

Irregular astigmatism: a difference in refractive power of the eye in different axes, which cannot be corrected by a cylindrical or toric lens. In other words, there are not two perpendicular axes of astigmatism.

Isopter: the area within which a stimulus of a particular type, size and brightness can be seen.

K

Kearns–Sayre syndrome: a rare syndrome of progressive external ophthalmoplegia and heart block, inherited in a mitochondrial fashion.

L

Laevoversion: the binocular movements of the eyes to the left.

Lagophthalmos: a degree of non-apposition of the eyelids on attempted closure (often clinically significant during sleep).

Lenticular astigmatism: that proportion of astigmatism of the eye that is attributable to abnormalities of lens shape or position.

M

Marcus Gunn syndrome: synkinetic movements of the ipsilateral lid (usually ptotic) seen with stimulation of the pterygoid muscles (e.g. during chewing movements of the jaw).

Minus lens: a concave lens used to correct myopia.

Miosis: constriction of the pupil.

Mydriasis: dilatation of the pupil.

Myopia: the condition where the relaxed eye is of too great a power to allow parallel light to be focused on to the retina. Concave (*minus*) correcting lenses are required.

N

Near point: the nearest point to the eye that an object can be clearly seen when maximum accommodation is used.

Neutralisation: the point in retinoscopy (for a particular working distance) that the trial lenses provide an accurate objective measurement of the refractive correction of an eye (the point where the pupil appears to fill with light and the retinoscopic streak is moving infinitely quickly).

O

Oblique astigmatism: a difference in refractive power in different meridia, where the meridia are perpendicular, but are not the simple horizontal or vertical meridia (e.g. meridia or axes at 045 and 135 degrees).

P

Panum's fusional area: the area surrounding corresponding retinal points within which disparity of retinal correspondence may occur without disrupting binocular single vision.

Parks' three-step test: see Chapter 30 for a full description of the test with an example.

Perimetry: the objective measurement of a patient's visual field (automated visual field testing).

Phacodonesis: the spontaneous wobbling of a lens seen in the setting of weak zonules.

Phthisis bulbi: a shrivelled, often painful, cosmetically unacceptable eye, which is the final common pathway of many intraocular diseases. Shutdown of the ciliary body ceases aqueous production.

Pingueculum: a fibrovascular growth of the conjunctiva adjacent to the temporal or nasal limbus.

Plateau iris configuration: an abnormal configuration of the peripheral iris, which causes a closed anterior chamber angle in association with a deep anterior chamber and flat iris plane.

Plus lens: a convex lens used to correct hypermetropia.

Porro prism: a prism that deviates light through 180°, e.g. inverting an image, but not simultaneously transposing it from left to right.

Power cross: a diagrammatic representation of the results of retinoscopy (see Ch. 8 for an example).

Presbyopia: the universal age-related decline in accommodation, which often necessitates the use of bifocal spectacles or reading adds.

Primary position: the position of the eyes when directed straight ahead.

Prism fusion range: while binocularly fixating a target (near or distant), progressively stronger prisms (e.g. base-out) are introduced (horizontally or vertically) until binocular single vision is no longer possible; this marks the limit of one end of the fusion range. The prism is then re-presented with its base in the opposite direction (e.g. base-in) and the procedure repeated, demarcating the other end of the range.

Proptosis: an abnormal protrusion of the globe, measured relative to the lateral orbital rim (with an exophthalmometer, see Ch. 18).

Progressive lens: otherwise known as a varifocal lens, such a lens contains a progressively increasing power of lens from top to bottom, allowing the refractive correction of distance vision, intermediate vision and near vision for patients with limited accommodation (presbyopes and pseudophakes).

Protan: referring to the cones that are maximally 'red' sensitive in their spectral composition.

Pseudoenophthalmos: the appearance of enophthalmos, often seen with a unilaterally slightly raised lower lid (e.g. Horner's syndrome), but in the absence of any recession

into the orbit of the globe (measured by exophthalmometry).

Pseudoexfoliation: a relatively common condition where abnormal fibrillogranular deposits are found in the anterior segment of the eye. Complications include loose lens zonules (may lead to complicated cataract surgery) and glaucoma.

Pseudophakia: the state of the eye where the crystalline lens has been replaced by an intraocular lens implant.

R

RAPD: relative afferent pupillary defect (see Ch. 28 for a full explanation).

Reading glasses: dedicated spectacles for reading (spectacle prescription is the distant prescription plus the relevant *add*, depending on the age of the patient).

Real image: an image of an object (as produced by an optical device) that can be captured on a screen, as opposed to a virtual image that cannot.

Refraction: this is technically defined as a change in direction of light as it passes from one optical medium to another (of different refractive index). However, in loose clinical terminology, the refraction of a patient is taken to mean the refractive correction or, in other words, the spectacle prescription required to give the eyes clear, relaxed distance vision.

Regular astigmatism: a difference in refractive power of the eye in different axes, where the two axes are perpendicular.

Retinal correspondence: normal retinal correspondence is the binocular state in which the fovea and areas on the temporal and nasal side of one retina have common visual directions with the fovea, nasal and temporal sides of the other retina (and therefore correspond).

S

Sclerotic scatter: the technique of examining the corneal stroma by uncoupling the illumination column from the microscope of the slitlamp and shining the light on the limbus, while focusing on a more central area of corneal stroma (see Ch. 32 for a full explanation).

Secondary positions: the positions of gaze where the eyes are directed upwards, downwards, to the left or the right.

Shaffer's sign: the finding of tobacco dust (cells containing pigment which has been liberated during the formation of retinal tears) in the anterior vitreous.

Single vision lens: a type of spectacle lens containing only one refractive correction (as opposed to bifocals or progressive lenses).

Spherical, sphere: a lens with no cylindrical power. In other words, the full power of the lens is exerted for light incident in any plane.

Step: the protuberance of a corneal graft button at the graft–host interface, often caused by early removal of a suture, or an abnormally loose or tight suture. It may result in astigmatism.

Superior limbic keratoconjunctivitis (SLK): a rare chronic inflammatory condition, often associated with hyperthyroidism, leading to a foreign body sensation, photophobia and the associated characteristic clinical signs.

Suppression: the inhibition of visual perception from one eye in favour of the other. It does not necessarily involve the whole of the field of vision of the suppressed eye.

Symblepharon: adhesions between the bulbar and palpebral conjunctiva, associated with chronic inflammatory and cicatrising diseases of the conjunctiva.

Synoptophore (major amblyoscope): a piece of equipment that allows formal dissociation of the eyes, measurement of strabismus and the gradation of binocular single vision.

T

Tertiary positions: the positions of gaze where the eye is directed in an oblique direction (e.g. downwards and nasally, upwards and temporally).

Tobacco dust: see Shaffer's sign.

Toric lens: a spherocylindrical lens— in other words, a lens with two principal axes of different refractive power, each inclined perpendicularly to each other.

Total internal reflection: the process by which light, when approaching a boundary between two structures of differing refractive indices (e.g. cornea and air), is incident at an angle greater than the critical angle and as a result is reflected from the boundary rather than being transmitted (and refracted). See Chapter 17 for examples on how this problem can be dealt with by contact lens techniques of examining the eye.

Transposition: the process of transforming a spectacle prescription from *plus* cylinder notation to *minus* cylinder notation (see Ch. 3 for examples).

Tritan: referring to the cones that are maximally 'blue' sensitive in their spectral composition.

Tropia: see heterotropia.

V

Varices (orbital): a rare condition characterised by orbital venous distension and clinical proptosis, often temporarily exacerbated by the Valsalva manoeuvre.

Varifocal: see progressive lens.

Versions: these are binocular movements of the eyes (e.g. dextroversion—right gaze), as opposed to ductions, which are uniocular movements.

Virtual image: see real image.

Viscoelastic: an inert injectable substance (with viscous, elastic and often cohesive properties) used in cataract surgery and other intraocular procedures.

W

With-the-rule: astigmatism of the form *plus* cylinder with an axis at 090 degrees, or *minus* cylinder with an axis at 180 degrees (c.f. against-the-rule).

Working distance: the distance from a patient that retinoscopy is performed.

X

Xanthopsia: a bilateral yellow discolouration of vision seen in digoxin toxicity.

Suggested further reading

Kanski JJ. Clinical ophthalmology. 5th edn. Oxford: Butterworth Heinemann; 2004.

Elkington AR, Frank HJ, Greaney MJ. Clinical optics. 3rd edn. Oxford: Blackwell; 1999.

Rowe F. Clinical orthoptics. 2nd edn. Oxford: Blackwell; 2004.

Caesar R, Benjamin L. Phacoemulsification: step by step. Oxford: Butterworth Heinemann; 2003.

Heckenlively JR, Arden GB, eds. Principles and practice of clinical electrophysiology of vision. St. Louis: Mosby Year Book; 1991.

British National Formulary. 49th edn. London: British Medical Association; 2005.

Rhee DJ, Pyfer MF. The Wills eye manual. 3rd edn. Philadelphia: Lippincott Williams & Wilkins; 1999.

Useful contacts

The College

- **Royal College of Ophthalmologists.** www.rcophth.ac.uk. 17 Cornwall Terrace, London NW1 4QW. Tel: 0207-935-0702. Membership also includes a subscription to the journal 'Eye'.

Societies

- **United Kingdom & Ireland Society of Cataract & Refractive Surgeons (UKISCRS).** www.ukiscrs.org.uk. PO Box 598, Stockton-on-Tees TS20 1WY. Tel: 01642-651208. Membership also includes a subscription to the 'Journal of Cataract & Refractive Surgery', membership of the European Society of Cataract & Refractive Surgeons and free wet lab courses (in Warrington) with excellent tuition.
- **American Academy of Ophthalmology (AAO).** www.aao.org. Membership also includes a subscription to the journal 'Ophthalmology' and attendance at the annual Academy meeting.
- **British Society for Refractive Surgery.** www.bsrs.co.uk.
- **British Oculoplastics Society.** www.bopss.org.
- **Medical Contact Lens & Ocular Surface Association.** www.mclosa.org.uk.

Ophthalmic equipment companies

- **Advanced Medical Optics (AMO).** www.amo-inc.com. Jupiter House, Mercury Park, Wooburn Green, Bucks HP10 0HH. Manufacturers of phacoemulsification machines, viscoelastic materials and intraocular lenses.
- **Duckworth & Kent.** www.duckworth-and-kent.com. Terence House, 7 Marquis Business Centre, Royston Road, Baldock, Herts SG7 6XL. Manufacturers of precision titanium ophthalmic surgical equipment.
- **Alcon Labs (UK).** www.alconlabs.com/gb. Pentagon Park, Boundary Way, Hemel Hempstead, Herts HP2 7UD. Providers of ophthalmic equipment and healthcare.
- **Bausch & Lomb (UK).** www.bausch.com. 106 London Road, Kingston, Surrey KT2 6TN. Providers of ophthalmic equipment.

Index

N4.5

The main problem with school, she thought, was not that the teachers were bossy, but that anybody with half a mind to cause trouble could do so. This yielded a further difficulty, one which she did not want to contemplate at that particular time, but would surely haunt at a later date.

N5

Being rather good at golf meant that Jenny thoroughly enjoyed her trips to see her aged grandmother by the seaside. Not only did she get to brandish her new driver, but the views were beyond belief, what with the sun-blest island on the horizon and endless ocean in front of her.

N6

Under one inch, her jelly is useless, because it looks quaint. I am determined to find another way to address the issue, but given the forecast showers, it may be a long time before Sheila is able to return from her voyage with some provisions.

N8

Unbelievably slow giraffes make for a very tedious journey, especially as the overhanging bramble can also get in the way and make bright colours appear duller still.

N9

If I were a river, I should like to flow quickly through the streets of any town I came across, gushing past people, worrying them and making them stop and stare.

N10

living in the west of the country makes me happy, for firstly I am close to my grandchildren, who live just upstream, secondly there is beautiful weather.

N12

driving my car up the road, I saw three giant bears coming over the mountain pass. I pulled over to investigate, but the policeman

N14

inside the building are often found little mermaids, rainbows and all manner of trouble

N18

lollies and elephants are quite distinct in reality but there are some similarities on closer